Foreword

I am honored to offer this short introduction to an important new project from Dr. Denis Cortese, Robert Smoldt and colleagues. This foreword gives me a rare and perhaps curious opportunity to draw a connection between two very different moments in my life, and, as I do so, it gives me an opportunity also to express my respect and esteem. Let me explain:

The first moment: from 1992 to 1995, I worked in Tokyo at the investment banking firm of JP Morgan & Co, eventually serving as a Managing Director. During these years, I grew in respect and esteem for my talented Japanese colleagues and for the remarkable accomplishments of Japanese society in so many ways.

The second moment: I currently serve as chair of the board of Catholic Health Initiatives ("CHI"), which is one of the largest healthcare organizations in the United States, with more than 90 hospitals across the United States and with assets of some $ 21 Billion. Robert Smoldt, one of the authors of the following important study, was a colleague of mine on the CHI board, and I have come to respect the very important work he and his colleague Denis Cortese are accomplishing in the United States in helping us to reflect on how our healthcare system can be improved.

The connection between these moments: What connection can there possibly be between these two very different moments? Well, perhaps quite a lot. During my years at JP Morgan in Japan, our business and Japan's economy were undergoing massive change. We understood very well that we too had to change in order to continue to thrive. Therefore, we were always eager to study new ideas and to compare best practices.

In the present moment, the world of healthcare is also undergoing dramatic change, certainly in the United States; and, just as in my investment banking days, we are very aware that we must change the way we do healthcare, and that we must be open to new ideas and approaches. It is well known, for example, that the U.S. spends significantly more per capita and a higher percentage of the Gross Domestic Product (GDP) on healthcare than other developed nations, yet our health outcomes and access to care remain disparate and inconsistent. Is it possible that similar variability in quality and cost of care exists in other countries? Can we in the U.S. learn by understanding better the approach and system of nations like Japan? Might our Japanese colleagues also learn by comparing their experience and outcomes with ours in the United States? More generally, could there be some common lessons for providers and policy makers around the world on improving the value of healthcare delivery (better patient outcomes using fewer resources per patient)?

These are some of the very interesting questions that Dr. Cortese and their colleagues are raising in their important and provocative new work. The following publication aims to examine potential opportunities for healthcare system improvement by evaluating patient outcomes and related expenditures for total joint replacements from a representative group of hospitals in Japan. Combining these empirical observations with an examination of system incentives, in particular those around provider reimbursement, the authors suggest that if payers of healthcare services were to pay for value, we would all be more likely to get it. The authors also provide a set of recommendations on how to begin on this road to pay for value, recommendations that are as applicable and relevant to the U.S. as they are to Japan. Healthcare professionals and policy makers would definitely benefit from considering this point of view.

Chris Lowney

September 2015

Chris Lowney chairs the board of Catholic Health Initiatives, one of the largest US healthcare/hospital systems. He also has experience with the Japanese healthcare system. Chris served as a Managing Director of J.P. Morgan & Co in Tokyo, New York, Singapore and London. He is a popular speaker who has lectured in more than two-dozen countries.

Preface

The aim of this publication is to provide some evidence supporting the implementation of an Expanded Diagnosis Related Group payment model, as a first step toward the establishment of high-value healthcare delivery systems, characterized by better patient outcomes and more sustainable spending trends.

In our analysis, we chose to focus on the U.S. and the Japanese healthcare systems because of the inherent differences and similarities between the two systems. For example, unlike the U.S., Japan ranks highly in many international comparisons of health systems and health costs per capita are significantly lower. Japan also provides universal healthcare coverage to its citizens, something the U.S. is still trying to accomplish. At the same time, the majority of healthcare providers in both countries work within a fee-for-service system and in 2003, Japan introduced the Diagnosis Procedure Combination (DPC), a case-mix based, per-diem graduated payment system which has some similarities to the DRG system in the U.S.

We felt that by taking a compare and contrast approach, we might be able to identify some common lessons for providers and policy makers in both countries, that would in turn help shape the overarching strategy for healthcare system improvement.

Denis A. Cortese, MD; Natalie Landman, PhD; Robert K. Smoldt, MBA; Sachiko Watanabe, RN, MHSA, MAE; Aki Yoshikawa, PhD

September 2015

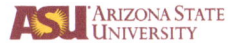 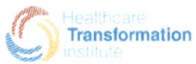 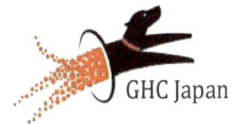

Table of contents

IN SEARCH OF HIGHER VALUE IN MEDICINE IN JAPAN AND THE U.S.

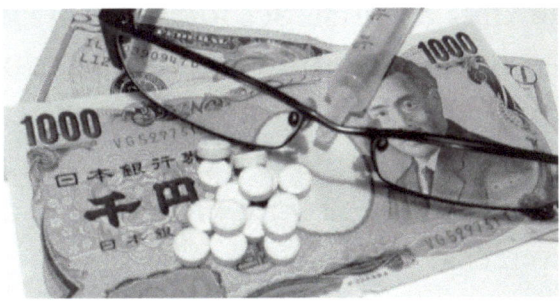

Denis A. Cortese, MD; Natalie Landman, PhD; Robert K. Smoldt, MBA; Sachiko Watanabe, RN, MHSA, MAE; Aki Yoshikawa, PhD

September 2015

Executive Summary

"Price is what you pay. Value is what you get."
- Warren Buffet

"Value – neither an abstract ideal nor a code word for cost reduction – should define the framework for performance improvement in healthcare. Rigorous, disciplined measurement and improvement of value is the best way to drive system progress."

- Michael E. Porter, Ph.D.

Source: Porter, Michael, E. (2010). What is Value in Health Care? *New England Journal of Medicine*, 363: 2477-2481.

Value can be defined and measured

$$\text{Value} = \frac{\textbf{Quality (Outcomes, Safety, Service)*}}{\textbf{Total Cost**}}$$

*Quality may include patient outcomes (e.g., mortality, faster return to work or functionality, readmission), safety (e.g., fewer complications, less rework), service (e.g., access to care, patient satisfaction). It may mean readiness or productivity in different groups, e.g., individual, employee, workforce, military, student.

**Total Cost may be spending over a defined time for a particular patient, a condition, a population, or a payer.

Source: 1) Smoldt RK, Cortese DA. Pay-for-performance or pay for value? *Mayo Clinic Proceedings*. Mayo Clinic 1 February 2007 (volume 82 issue 2 pages 210-213 DOI: 10.4065/82.2.210); 2) Porter ME. What is value in health care? *N Eng J Med*. 2010; 363: 2477-2481: http://www.nejm.org/doi/full/10.1056/NEJMp1011024 Accessed October 7, 2013; 3) Porter ME, Lee TH. The strategy that will fix health care. Harvard Business Review (2013): http://hbr.org/2013/10/the-strategy-that-will-fix-health-care/ar/1. Accessed October 7, 2013; 4) Fisher E, Sutherland J, Radley D. Dartmouth Medical School analysis of data from a 20% national sample of Medicare beneficiaries. *Commonwealth Fund*. National Scorecard on U.S. Health System Performance, 2011. Institute of Medicine. New data on geographic variation. 2011: http://www.iom.edu/Activities/HealthServices/GeographicVariation/Data-Resources.aspx

When value is measured, it is not unusual to find variability in quality and costs

- In fact, in 2010 the Organization for Economic Co-operation and Development (OECD) released a report analyzing the value of healthcare being delivered across and within its member nations.
- Among their key findings:
  - "...there is room in all countries surveyed to improve the effectiveness of their health care spending," and
  - "...there is no health care system that performs systematically better in delivering cost-effective health care."

Source: OECD 2010, "Health care systems: Getting more value for money", OECD Economics Department Policy Notes, No. 2.

So what are we striving for?

Our goal is straightforward:

Highest-value healthcare delivery = Better quality at lower costs

And how do we start?

- Change the existing healthcare provider financial incentives and start paying for value.
    - Specifically, as a valuable step in this journey, both the U.S. and Japan should move to an Extended DRG (EDRG) – one bundled payment that includes all the costs of hospital and physician services from the time of admission to a set date post admission.
    - We believe that this mechanism will serve as a forcing function on the path to a high-value care delivery system, one characterized by higher quality and lower resource utilization.

7

Key steps for establishing EDRGs in Japan

1. Replace the current payment system with a DRG-like classification.
2. Define bundles to include the full breadth of medical services associated with a given DRG for a pre-defined period of time (e.g., 90 days).
3. Establish a single payment amount for each bundle (using reality-based pricing).
4. Define target quality metrics and institute a quality withhold.
5. Require all hospitals to participate in the new payment system.

8

Where to start?

- Start with the top 3-5 most expensive conditions or procedures (e.g., total joints).
- Improve effectiveness and efficiency for these conditions or procedures based on quality and costs over time.
- Once completed, move on to the next most expensive set of DRGs.

Outline

1. The Japanese healthcare system: Challenges and opportunities
2. Practice variation in Japan: Total joint replacements
3. Practice variation in the U.S.
4. Summary and Recommendations

At first glance, Japan IS the healthcare system to emulate

- Japan ranks positively in many international comparisons of health systems in terms of health outcomes.

- Universal health insurance that provides basic access to healthcare services has been in place since 1961.

- The Japanese spend less on healthcare than other developed nations.

Japan ranks highly on mortality amenable to healthcare among developed nations

Mortality amenable to healthcare among OECD nations (2002-2003)
Deaths per 100,000 population

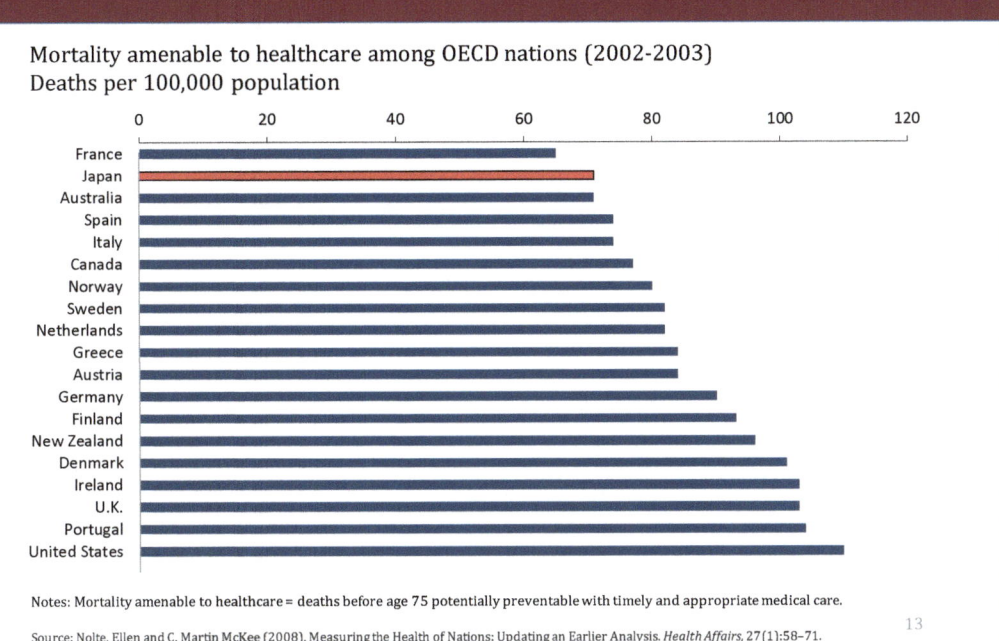

Notes: Mortality amenable to healthcare = deaths before age 75 potentially preventable with timely and appropriate medical care.

Source: Nolte, Ellen and C. Martin McKee (2008). Measuring the Health of Nations: Updating an Earlier Analysis. *Health Affairs*, 27(1):58–71.

13

Virtually all Japanese citizens and residents have health insurance coverage

- Japan began its quest for universal healthcare coverage with the passage of the Health Insurance Act of 1922.

- This formidable goal was reached in 1961 through a combination of employer- and community-based plans.

- Although the specifics of coverage have evolved over the years, today, nearly all Japanese people are covered by the public health insurance system through >3,400 plans.

Source: 1) Ikegami et al. 2011. Japanese universal health coverage: evolution, achievements, and challenges. *The Lancet*, 378:1106-15; 2) International profiles of healthcare systems, 2014. The Commonwealth Fund.

14

Japan spends significantly less on healthcare per capita than other nations

Total health expenditures per capita (2012)
PPP$

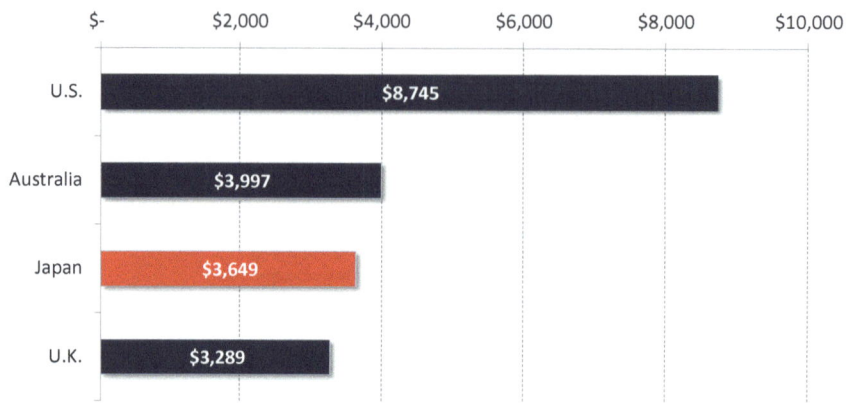

	$-	$2,000	$4,000	$6,000	$8,000	$10,000

- U.S. — $8,745
- Australia — $3,997
- Japan — $3,649
- U.K. — $3,289

Notes: PPP $ = purchasing power parity, the amount of money needed to purchase the same goods and services in two different countries; used to calculate an implicit foreign exchange rate.

Source: OECD Health Data 2014 (accessed September 16, 2014), http://stats.oecd.org/index.aspx?DataSetCode=HEALTH_STAT

15

But not all that glitters is gold

- Access to healthcare services does not always translate into high-value care:
  - "Patients can nearly always see a doctor within a day. But they must often wait hours for a three-minute consultation....The Japanese are only a quarter as likely as the Americans or French to suffer a heart attack, but twice as likely to die if they do."[1]
- Allocation of medical resources leaves a lot to be desired:
  - "A vivid example: Japan's emergency rooms, which every year turn away tens of thousands who need care"[2]

Source: 1) Health care in Japan: Not all Smiles. *The Economist.* http://www.economist.com/node/21528660. 2011. Accessed July 29, 2014; 2) Improving Japan's health care system. *McKinsey Quarterly,* March 2009. Accessed September 16, 2014.

16

But not all that glitters is gold (cont'd)

- There are significant delays in the introduction of new treatments, devices and vaccines.[1]
- There is virtually no control over demand and supply of healthcare:
  - "...patients are free to consult any provider...at any time, without proof of medical necessity...Physicians may practice wherever they chose, in any area of medicine."[2]

Source: 1) Shibuya et al. 2011. Future of Japan's system of good health at low cost with equity: beyond universal coverage. *The Lancet*, 378:1265-73: 2) Improving Japan's health care system. *McKinsey Quarterly*, March 2009. Accessed September 16, 2014.

Organization of the Japanese healthcare system promotes inefficiency

Hospital beds per 1,000 population (2012)*

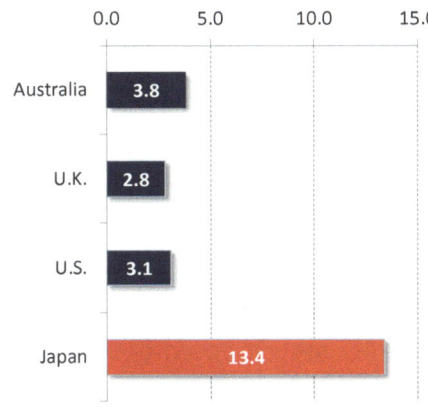

CT scanners per million population (2012)*

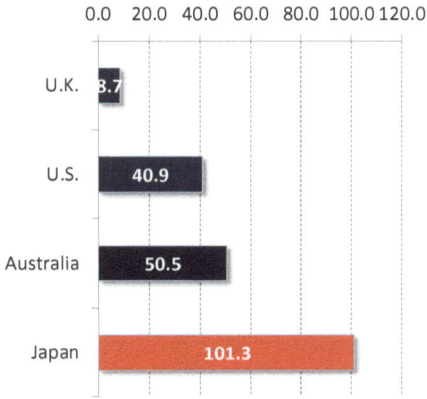

System inefficiencies are exacerbated by demographic and economic trends

- Japan needs a strong workforce to finance its healthcare system since 38.1% of the program's costs come from general government revenues, and 48.5% are paid via payroll taxes.
- Yet it is faced with a rapidly aging population and a changing structure of the economy:
  - The proportion of Japanese 65 years and older is projected to reach 30% by 2020 (and account for 66% of total healthcare expenditures),
  - As a result of competition, deregulation, and changing corporate priorities more workers in Japan are being hired on a temporary, part-time or contract basis.

Source: 1) Ikegami et al. 2011. Japanese universal health coverage: evolution, achievements, and challenges. *The Lancet*, 378:1106-15; 2) International profiles of healthcare systems, 2014. The Commonwealth Fund; 3) Xu and Yamada. 2013. Financing Health Care in Japan: A Rapidly Aging Population and the Dilemma of Reforms. http://www3.grips.ac.jp/~minchunghsu/JPHI201305_Hsu_Yamada.pdf. Accessed May 22, 2015.

So what can be done to get back on track?

- Japan is making strides in the right direction with its intent to change medical center reimbursement from per-diem to bundled payments.
- In a Commonwealth article, Zezza, Guterman and Smith have accurately noted that in this approach "payment levels must be carefully calibrated to ensure providers financial viability while providing incentives to reduce costs and safeguards to ensure high quality."
- Utilizing total joint replacement data from over 500 Japanese hospitals, this publication explores a method for bundled payments that could serve as a valuable step in moving the healthcare delivery system toward high-value care.

Source: Zezza, M; Guterman, S; Smith, J. The Bundled Payment for Care Improvement Initiative: Achieving High-Value Care with a Single Payment. The Commonwealth Fund Blog, January 7, 2012. http://www.commonwealthfund.org/Blog/2012/Jan/Bundled-Payment-for-Care-Improvement.aspx; Accessed April 24, 2014.

Japanese total joint data presents a great case study

- In order to effectively determine the quality and cost implications these payment models incentivize within Japanese hospitals, we performed an analysis on value metrics around total joint replacements.

- We were especially interested in the Japanese total joint data because in both Japan and the United States the total knee replacement aggregate procedure cost is one of the highest among procedures covered by payers, thus making total joint replacements an excellent medical category for this study.

Source: 1) Anderson, Gerard, Ikegami, Naoki. (2011). How Can Japan's DPC Inpatient Hospital Payment System Be Strengthened? Lessons from the U.S. Medicare Prospective System. *Center for Strategic and International Studies.* http://csis.org/publication/how-can-japans-dpc-inpatient-hospital-payment-system-be-strengthened; 2) AHRQ. Weighted national estimates from HCUP National Inpatient Sample (NIS), 2012 Total number of weighted discharges in the U.S. based on HCUP NIS = 36,484,846. http://hcupnet.ahrq.gov/HCUPnet.jsp

Japanese total joint data presents a great case study for the U.S. (cont'd)

- The comparison with Japan is particularly compelling as the majority of healthcare providers in Japan function in a fee-for-service payment structure, where prices are set by government entities – not unlike the experience of the majority of U.S. providers.

- Moreover, in 2003, Japan introduced the Diagnosis Procedure Combination (DPC), a case-mix based, per-diem graduated payment system that uses a 14-digit classification code to identify major disease categories as well as treatments and procedures, which has some similarities to the DRG system in the U.S.

Source: Anderson, Gerard, Ikegami, Naoki. (2011). How Can Japan's DPC Inpatient Hospital Payment System Be Strengthened? Lessons from the U.S. Medicare Prospective System. *Center for Strategic and International Studies.* http://csis.org/publication/how-can-japans-dpc-inpatient-hospital-payment-system-be-strengthened

Outline

1. The Japanese healthcare system: Challenges and opportunities
2. Practice variation in Japan: Total joint replacements
3. Practice variation in the U.S.
4. Summary and Recommendations

Introduction

- All analyses were carried out on data aggregated at the hospital level from acute care facilities in the Global Health Consulting Japan (GHC Japan) hospital discharge database.

- GHC Japan, a hospital consulting firm, provides a variety of consulting services to over 800 Japanese hospitals paid on the DPC per-diem methodology.

- Although DPC paid facilities constitute about one fifth of the total number of hospitals in Japan, DPC facilities tend to be the larger hospitals. As a result, about half (51.7%) of all hospital beds are paid under the DPC system.[1] In turn, the GHC Japan database spans eight geographical regions and accounts for 54% of all DPC facilities.

Source: Anderson, Gerard, Ikegami, Naoki. (2011). How Can Japan's DPC Inpatient Hospital Payment System Be Strengthened? Lessons from the U.S. Medicare Prospective System. *Center for Strategic and International Studies.*
http://csis.org/publication/how-can-japans-dpc-inpatient-hospital-payment-system-be-strengthened

Total Knee Replacements (TKR)

TKR methods and data overview

- We identified 549 hospitals in the GHC Japan hospital discharge database that performed at least one total knee replacement (TKR) between April 1 and December 31, 2012.

- All hospitals where data were collected for less than six months were excluded from our analysis.

- In addition, all cases of double-joint replacements were excluded, giving us a final sample size of **514 hospitals** and **11,289 TKR cases**.

- For comparisons with prior studies that examined total joint replacement, we annualized the number of total joint cases performed by a given hospital.

- These "estimated" case numbers for each facility are based on the number of cases observed over the period of data collection and assume a consistent rate of procedures across a 12-month period.

Table 1A: Summary metrics for TKR sample

	Mean	Median	Minimum	Maximum
Age	75.0	74.9		
Hospital characteristics (n=514)				
Data collection duration[a] (months)	8.5	9.0	6.0	9.0
Annual Estimated Hospital Volume[b]	31	20	1	381
Value metrics				
Complication Rate[c]	4.78%	2.20%	0.0%	100%
Average Hospital Revenue/TKR case[d] (dollars)	$19,192	$18,909	$14,049	$43,299
Length of Stay[e] (days)	28.9	27.9	11.5	144

[a]Data were collected for hospitals that performed at least one TKR between April and December 2012
[b]Data were collected for a 6-9 month period and annualized in order to give an estimated annual case load
[c]Post-operative complication rate is calculated for each facility and identified by the presence of one or more complication including surgical site infections, reoperation, post-op bleeding, post-op bed sores, post-op acute respiratory distress syndrome, pulmonary embolism, post-op septicemia, and in-hospital death
[d]Average hospital revenue is calculated by dividing the total DPC payments received by a facility by the total number of TKR cases performed at that facility for the duration of observation and weighted by the number of cases each facility performed
[e]Average length of stay is calculated as a weighted average across all facilities and includes the acute portion of hospitalization only
Note: All data were aggregated at the level of an individual hospital prior to analysis

Japanese hospitals have lower TKR case volumes than U.S. hospitals

- One of the first observations about our sample of 514 TKR performing hospitals was that the average number of TKRs performed is low = 31 cases annually (Table 1A).

- For comparison, only the top 10% of Japanese hospitals in our sample performed more cases than the bottom 10% in Florida (Table 2A).

- In fact, ~25% of the hospitals in our sample did fewer than 10 TKR cases per year (or fewer than one case per month), and ~90% of hospitals did fewer than 70 cases per year (Table 2A, Figure 1A).

- In comparison, 100% of the hospitals in Florida (for which we had data; n=155) performed at least 31 cases annually and 80% performed ≥ 90 cases each year.

Table 2A: Annual TKR cases per hospital, Japan vs. Florida

	Estimated annual Japan TKR cases (n=514) (Apr. 2012 – Mar. 2013)	Annual Florida TKR cases (n=155) (Oct. 2013 – Sept. 2014)
Average	31	272
Minimum	1	31
Maximum	381	1338
Percentile		
10th	4	61
20th	8	88
30th	11	135
40th	15	173
50th	20	201
60th	27	276
70th	36	339
80th	44	404
90th	67	529

Figure 1A: Distribution of TKR cases per hospital, Japan vs. Florida

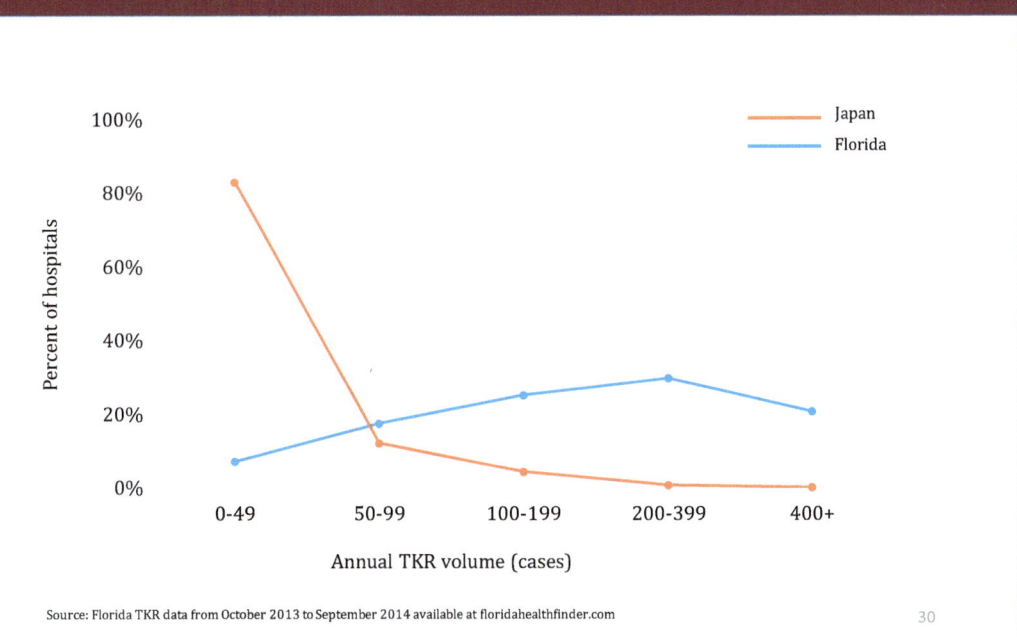

Volume of TKR procedures is correlated with patient complications

- We also observed the previously established correlation between low volume of procedures performed and higher patient complications.

- Figure 2A shows the distribution of post-operative complication rates as a function of the number of TKR cases performed at a given facility.

- It is clear that for this hospital data set, post-operative complication rates were higher among hospitals performing less than 70 TKR cases per year.

Figure 2A: TKR post-operative complication rate vs. estimated annual hospital volume

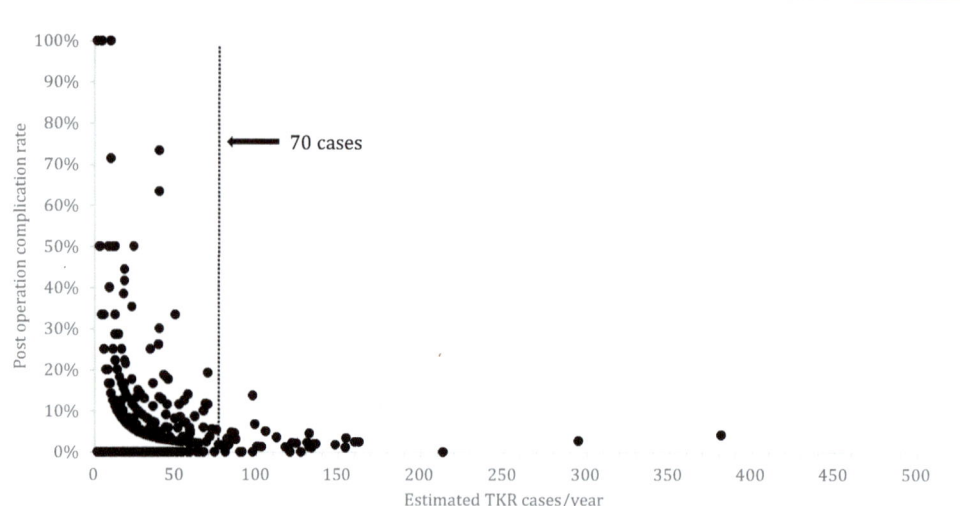

Data were collected from hospitals for a 6-9 month period. The number of cases were then annualized in order to give an estimated annual case load. Post-operative complication rate is calculated for each facility and identified by one or more complication including surgical site infections, reoperation, post-op bleeding, post-op bed sores, post-op acute respiratory distress syndrome, pulmonary embolism, post-op septicemia, and in-hospital death. 514 sample DPC hospitals displayed and each point is representative of one hospital.

We observed significant length of stay (LOS), as well as significant LOS variation

- The average Length of stay (LOS) for TKR was calculated as a weighted average across all facilities and includes the acute portion of hospitalization only.
- The weighted average LOS for total knee replacement was 28.9 days (Figure 3A).
- The median LOS for the TKR patients in our sample was 27.9 days.
- We observed wide variability among the hospitals, with more than a 10-fold difference between the hospital with the lowest LOS (11.5 days) and the hospital with the highest LOS (144 days).

Figure 3A: Distribution of length of stay (LOS) for TKR cases

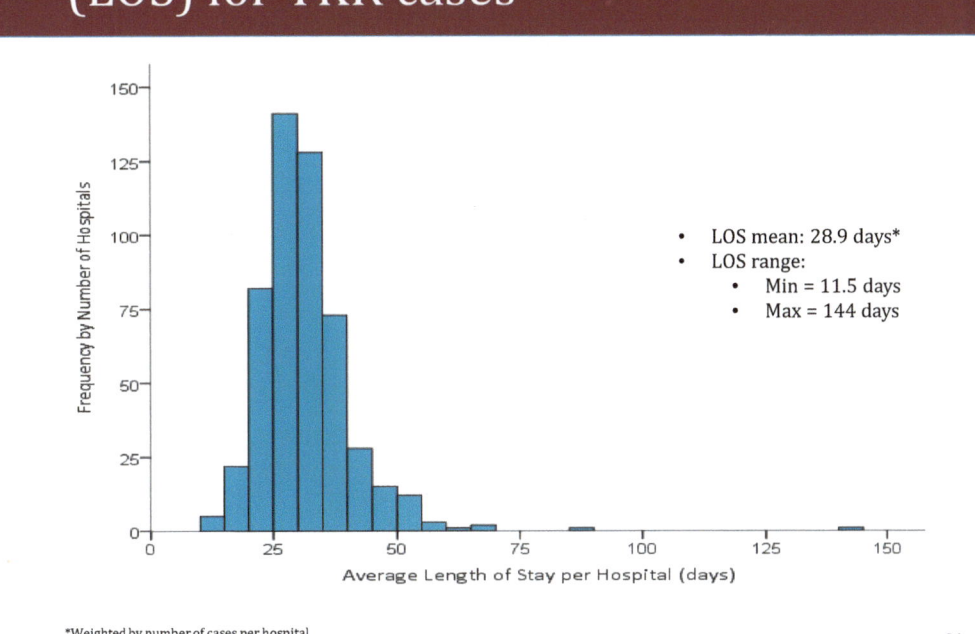

- LOS mean: 28.9 days*
- LOS range:
  - Min = 11.5 days
  - Max = 144 days

*Weighted by number of cases per hospital

Limited correlation observed between TKR LOS and post-operative complication rate

- It is feasible that the observed longer length of stays are a result of higher complication rates in our patient sample.
- To that end we ran a simple correlation between post-operative complication rates and LOS for each of the facilities in our sample.
- We calculated an R = 0.23, R^2 = 0.05 (p < 0.01) for TKR cases (Figure 4A).
- It is most interesting to note that even those hospitals that had no post-operative complications show a range of LOS from a minimum of 11.5 to a maximum of 144 days for TKR (Figure 5A).

Figure 4A: TKR LOS vs. post-operative complication rate

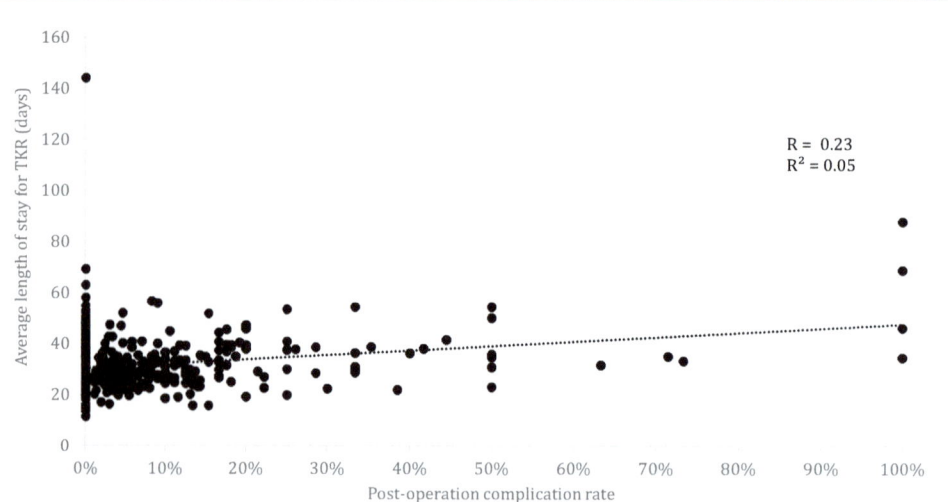

Average length of stay is calculated across all cases of TKR performed in a given facility and includes the acute portion of hospitalization only. Post-operative complication rate is calculated for each facility and identified by one or more complication including surgical site infections, reoperation, post-op bleeding, post-op bed sores, post-op acute respiratory distress syndrome, pulmonary embolism, post-op septicemia, and in-hospital death. 514 DPC sample hospitals displayed and each point is representative of one hospital.

Figure 5A: TKR LOS in hospitals with 0% post-operative complication rate

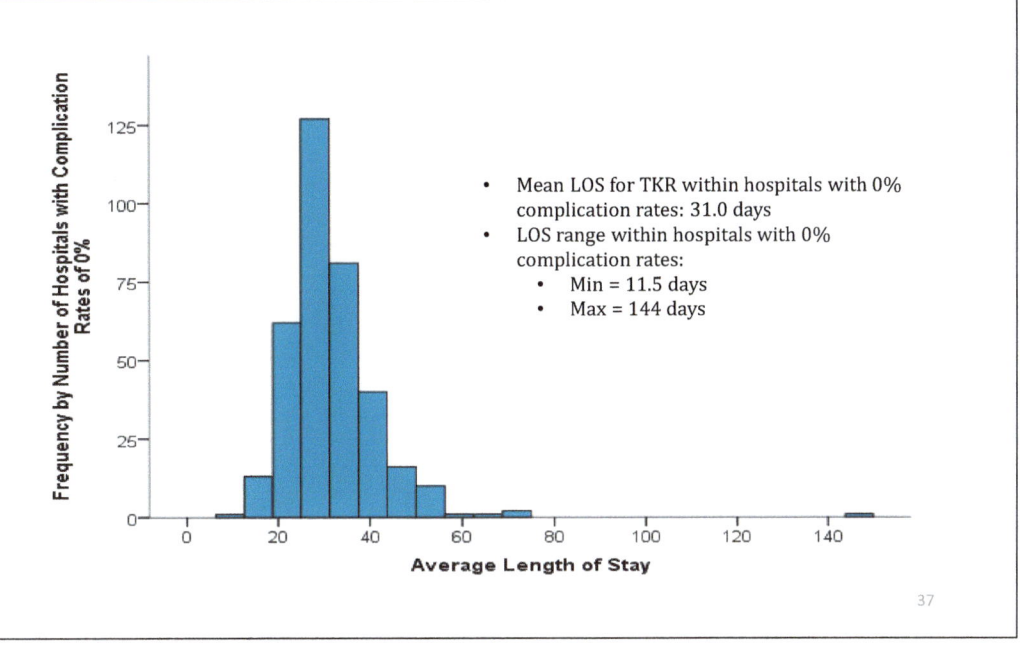

- Mean LOS for TKR within hospitals with 0% complication rates: 31.0 days
- LOS range within hospitals with 0% complication rates:
  - Min = 11.5 days
  - Max = 144 days

We also observed significant variability in TKR revenue among our sample hospitals

- The average revenue across all facilities was weighted by estimated annual case load per hospital. All figures are in USD.

- The mean revenue for all hospitals was $19,192 per TKR case (Figure 6A).

- Not surprisingly, due to the variance in LOS metrics and the per diem payment model, we also found a large variance in revenue among the hospitals, with the highest revenue hospital ($43,299) earning more than 3 times per case than the lowest revenue hospital ($14,049).

- Moreover, we found a significant correlation (R = 0.89 and R^2 = 0.79, p<0.01) between hospital LOS and hospital revenue for TKR as shown in Figure 7A.

Figure 6A: Distribution of TKR per case hospital revenue

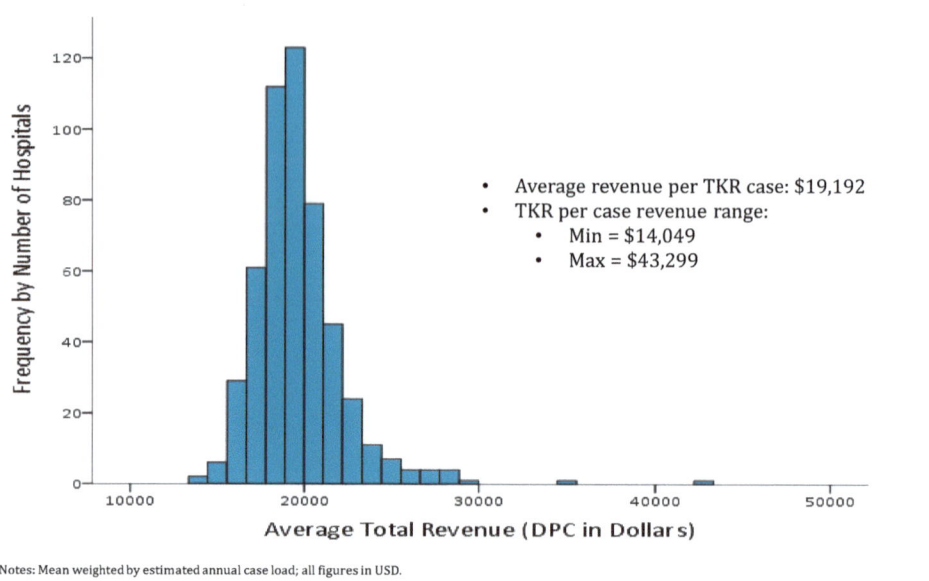

- Average revenue per TKR case: $19,192
- TKR per case revenue range:
  - Min = $14,049
  - Max = $43,299

Notes: Mean weighted by estimated annual case load; all figures in USD.

Figure 7A: TKR hospital revenue per case vs. LOS

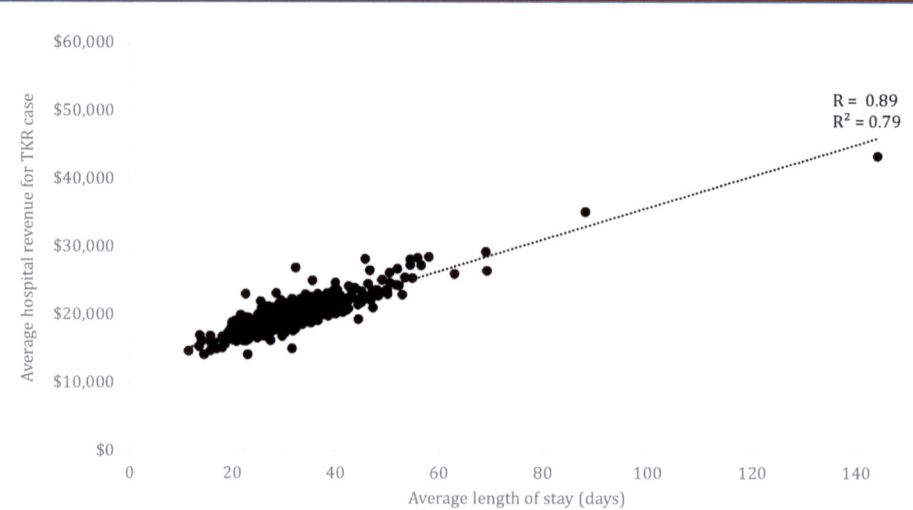

R = 0.89
R² = 0.79

Average length of stay is calculated across all cases of TKR performed in a given facility and includes the acute portion of hospitalization only. Average hospital revenue is calculated by dividing the total DPC payments received by a facility by the total number of cases performed at that facility for the duration of observation. 514 DPC sample hospitals displayed and each point is representative of one hospital.

No clear relationship between hospital revenue per case and post-operative complications

- In contrast to the strong correlation observed for hospital revenue and LOS, we calculated R = 0.25, R^2 = 0.06 (p < 0.01) for relationship between hospital revenue and post-operative complication rates.
- The average revenue per case is designated by the orange vertical line in Figure 8A and the orange horizontal line designates the average post-operative complication rate.
- Moreover, we found a large variation in revenue even for hospitals that had no post-surgical complications – from $14,049 to $43,299 per TKR case (Figure 9A).

Figure 8A: TKR post-operative complication rate vs. hospital revenue

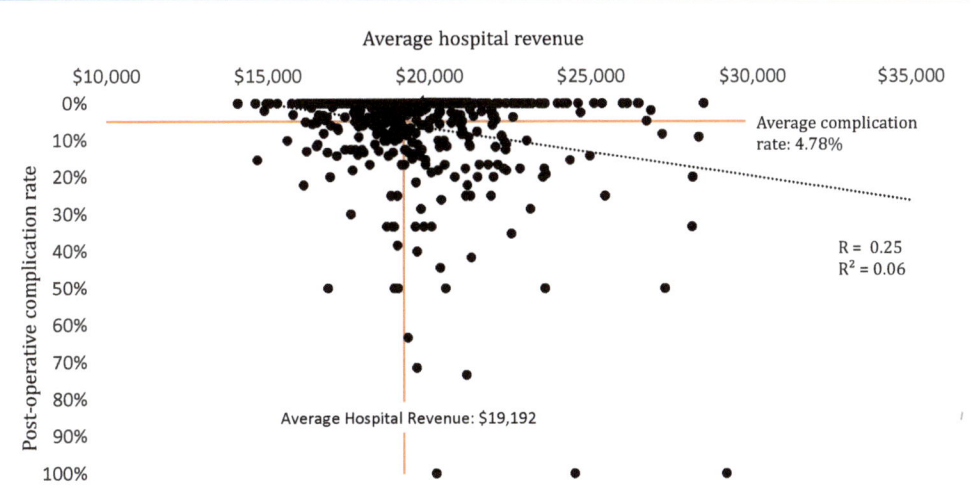

Post-operative complication rate is calculated for each facility and identified by one or more complication including surgical site infections, reoperation, post-op bleeding, post-op bed sores, post-op acute respiratory distress syndrome, pulmonary embolism, post-op septicemia, and in-hospital death. Average hospital revenue is calculated by dividing the total DPC payments received by a facility by the total number of cases performed at that facility for the duration of observation. Each point represents one hospital.

Figure 9A: Distribution of TKR revenue in facilities with 0% post-operative complication rate

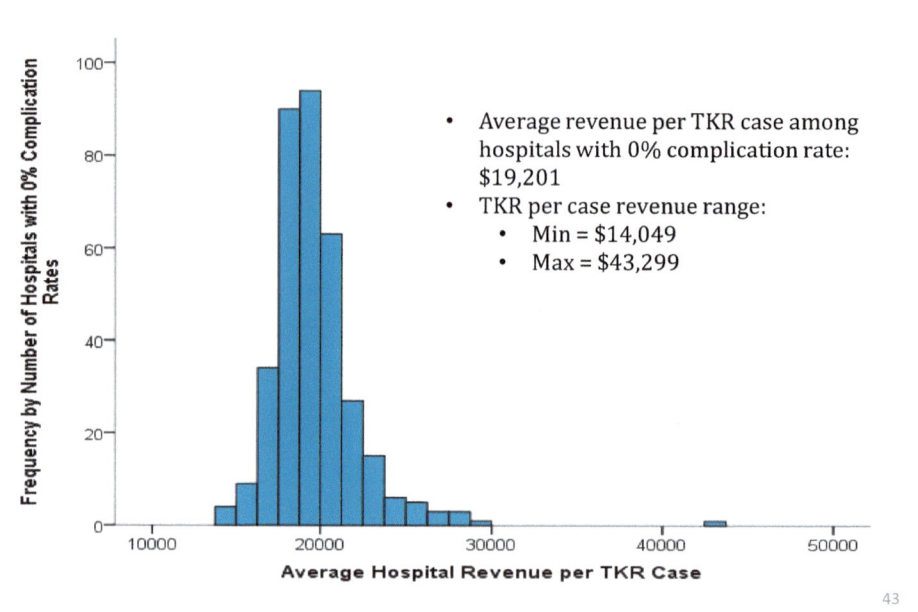

- Average revenue per TKR case among hospitals with 0% complication rate: $19,201
- TKR per case revenue range:
  - Min = $14,049
  - Max = $43,299

43

Total Hip Replacements (THR)

THR methods and data overview

- We identified 594 hospitals that performed at least one total hip replacement (THR) between April 1 and December 31, 2012.

- All hospitals where data were collected for less than six months were excluded from our analysis.

- In addition, all cases of double-joint replacements were excluded, giving us a final sample size **574 hospitals** and **12,006 THR cases**.

- For comparisons with prior studies that examined total joint replacement, we annualized the number of total joint cases performed by a given hospital.

- These "estimated" case numbers for each facility are based on the number of cases observed over the period of data collection and assume a consistent rate of procedures across a 12-month period.

Table 1B: Summary metrics for THR sample

	Mean	Median	Minimum	Maximum
Age	66.7	66.4		
Hospital characteristics (n=574)				
Data collection duration[a] (months)	8.9	9.0	6.0	9.0
Annual Estimated Hospital Volume[b]	28	15	1	457
Value metrics				
Complication Rate[c]	5.54%	2.70%	0.0%	100.0%
Average Hospital Revenue/THR case[d] (dollars)	$22,569	$22,204	$16,149	$57,034
Length of Stay[e] (days)	28.9	27.6	12.6	125

[a]Data were collected for hospitals that performed at least one THR between April and December 2012
[b]Data were collected for a 6-9 month period and annualized in order to give an estimated annual case load.
[c]Post-operative complication rate is calculated for each facility and identified by the presence of one or more complication including surgical site infections, reoperation, post-op bleeding, post-op bed sores, post-op acute respiratory distress syndrome, pulmonary embolism, post-op septicemia, and in-hospital death
[d]Average hospital revenue is calculated by dividing the total DPC payments received by a facility by the total number of THR cases performed at that facility for the duration of observation and weighted by the number of cases each facility performed
[e]Average length of stay is calculated as a weighted average across all facilities and includes the acute portion of hospitalization only
All data were aggregated at the level of an individual hospital prior to analysis

Japanese hospitals have lower THR procedure volumes than U.S. hospitals

- One of the first observations about our sample of 574 THR performing hospitals was that the average number of THRs is low = 28 cases annually (Table 1B).

- We also found that ~20% of hospitals in our sample performed 5 or fewer THR cases per year and ~90% of hospitals did 70 or fewer THRs annually (Table 2B).

- In contrast, every Florida hospital (for which we had data; n=160) performed at least 30 THRs and 80% of Florida hospitals performed >70 cases annually (Table 2B, Figure 1B).

- It is worth noting that both Japan and Florida experienced significant variability in the volume of cases between hospitals within their respective geographic regions.

Source: Florida TKR and THR data from October 2012 to September 2013 available at floridahealthfinder.com

Table 2B: Annual THR cases per hospital, Japan vs. Florida

	Estimated annual Japan THR cases (n=574) (Apr. 2012 – Mar. 2013)	Annual Florida THR cases (n=160) (Oct. 2013 – Sept. 2014)
Average	28	210
Minimum	1	30
Maximum	457	865
Percentile		
10th	3	52
20th	5	76
30th	8	94
40th	11	118
50th	15	156
60th	20	192
70th	27	253
80th	40	335
90th	68	443

Source: Florida THR data from October 2013 to September 2014 available at floridahealthfinder.com

Figure 1B: Distribution of THR cases per hospital, Japan vs. Florida

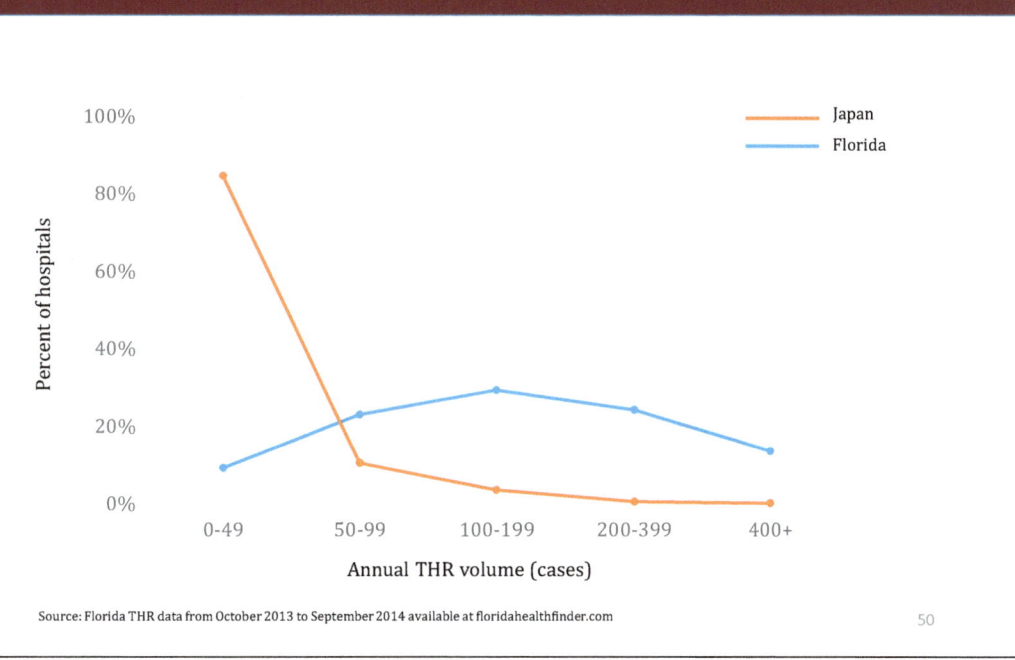

Source: Florida THR data from October 2013 to September 2014 available at floridahealthfinder.com

Volume of THR procedures is correlated with patient complications

- We also observed the previously established correlation between low volume of procedures performed and higher patient complications.
- Figure 2B shows the distribution of post-operative complication rates as a function of the number of THR cases performed at a given facility.
- It is clear that for this hospital data set, post-operative complication rates were higher among hospitals performing less than 70 THR cases per year.

51

Figure 2B: THR Post-operative complication rates vs. estimated annual hospital volume

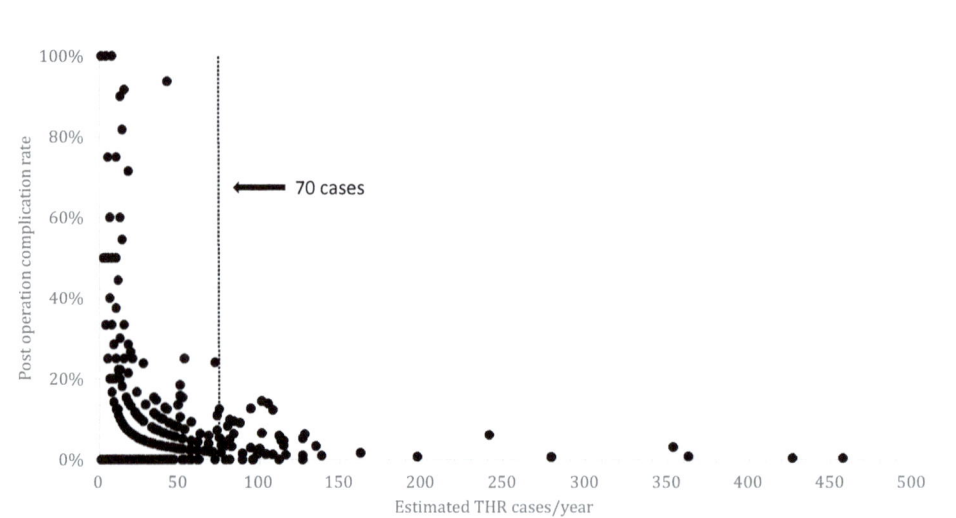

Data were collected from hospitals for a 6-9 month period. The number of cases were then annualized in order to give an estimated annual case load. Post-operative complication rate is calculated for each facility and identified by one or more complication including surgical site infections, reoperation, post-op bleeding, post-op bed sores, post-op acute respiratory distress syndrome, pulmonary embolism, post-op septicemia, and in-hospital death. 574 DPC sample hospitals displayed and each point is representative of one hospital.

52

We observed significant length of stay (LOS), as well as significant LOS variation

- The average length of stay (LOS) for THR was calculated as a weighted average across all facilities and includes the acute portion of hospitalization only.
- The weighted average LOS for THR was 28.9 days (Figure 3B).
- The median LOS for THR patients in our sample was 27.6 days.
- We again observed significant variability among the hospitals, with a nearly 10-fold difference between the hospital with the lowest LOS (12.6 days) and the hospital with the highest LOS (125 days).

Figure 3B: Distribution of length of stay (LOS) for THR cases

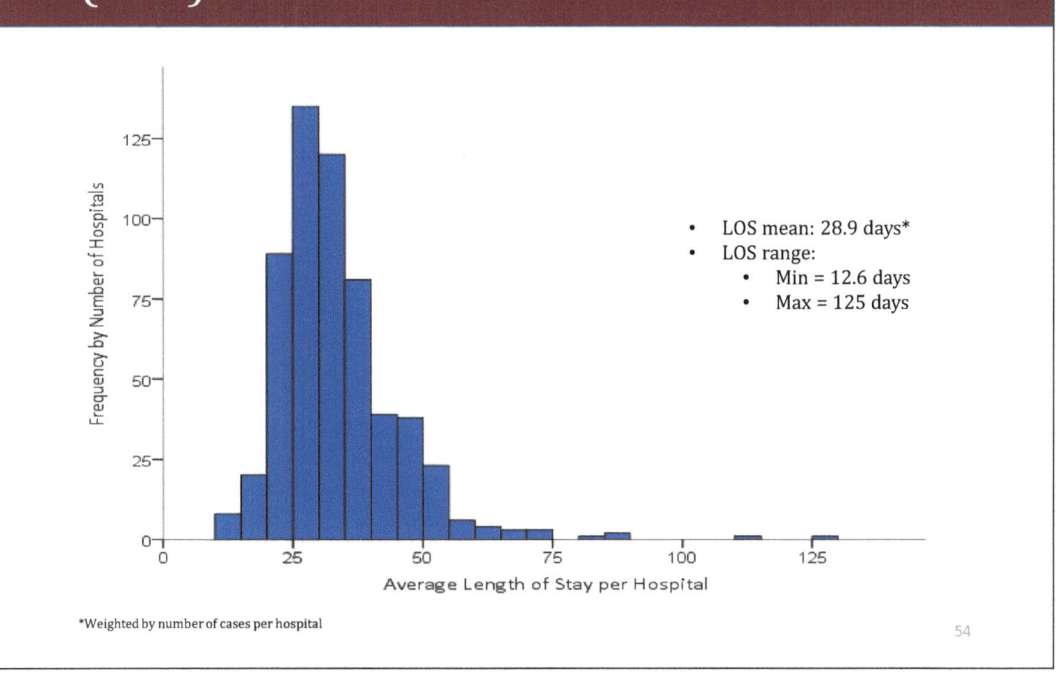

- LOS mean: 28.9 days*
- LOS range:
  - Min = 12.6 days
  - Max = 125 days

*Weighted by number of cases per hospital

Limited correlation between THR LOS and post-operative complication rate

- It is feasible that the observed longer length of stays are a result of higher complication rates in our patient sample.
- To that end we ran a simple correlation between post-operative complication rates and LOS for each of the facilities in our sample.
- We calculated an R=0.12, $R^2 = 0.01$ (p < 0.01) for THR cases (Figure 4B).
- It is most interesting to note that even those hospitals that had no post-operative complications show a range of LOS from a minimum of 12.6 to a maximum of 125 days for THR (Figure 5B).

Figure 4B: THR hospital LOS vs. post-operative complication rate

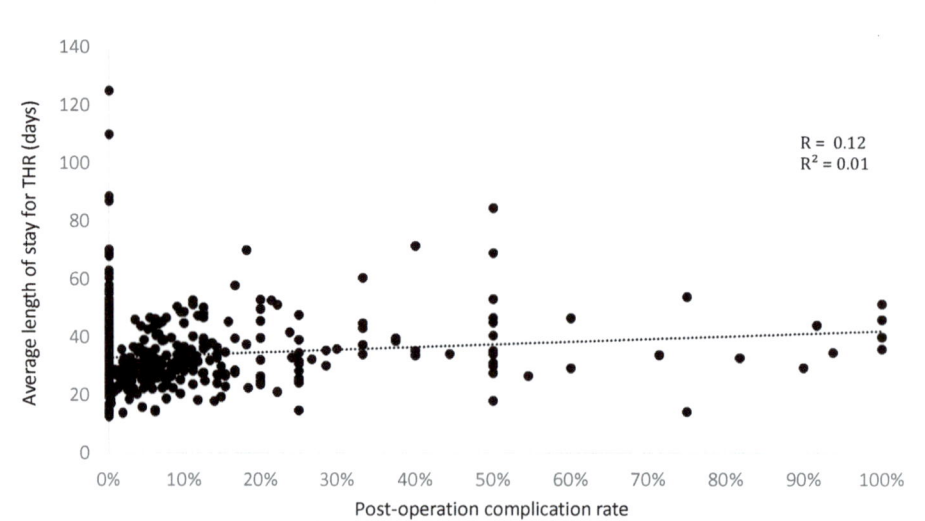

Average length of stay is calculated across all cases of THR performed in a given facility and includes the acute portion of hospitalization only. Post-operative complication rate is calculated for each facility and identified by one or more complication including surgical site infections, reoperation, post-op bleeding, post-op bed sores, post-op acute respiratory distress syndrome, pulmonary embolism, post-op septicemia, and in-hospital death. 574 DPC sample hospitals displayed and each point is representative of one hospital.

Figure 5B: Distribution of THR LOS in hospitals with 0% complication rates

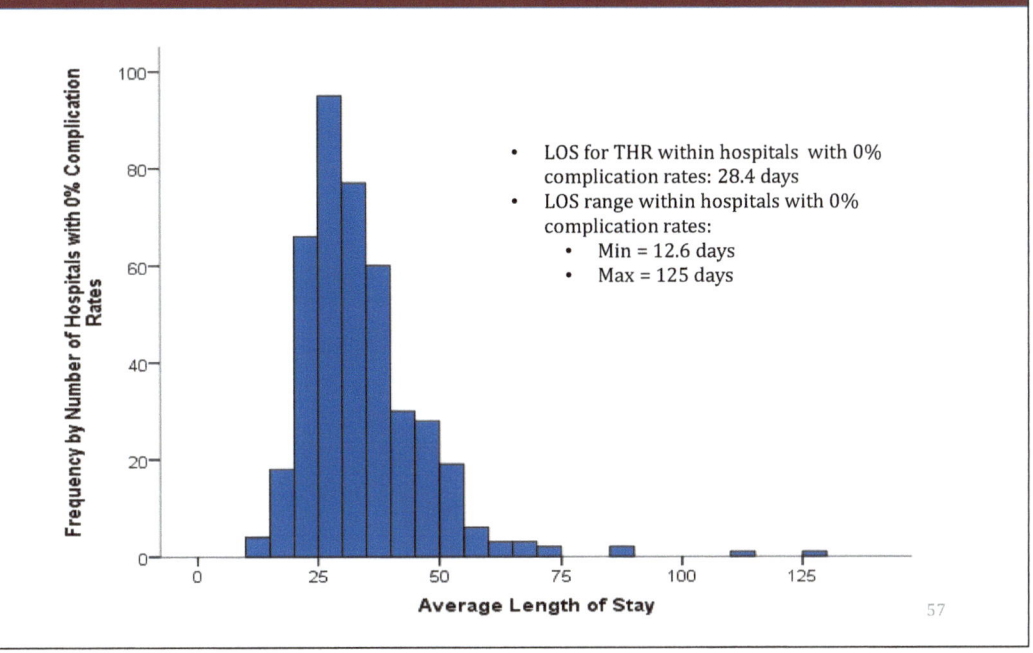

- LOS for THR within hospitals with 0% complication rates: 28.4 days
- LOS range within hospitals with 0% complication rates:
  - Min = 12.6 days
  - Max = 125 days

We also observed significant variability in THR revenue among our sample hospitals

- The average revenue across all facilities was weighted by estimated annual case load per hospital. All figures are in USD.
- The mean THR per case revenue for all hospitals was $22,569 (Figure 6B).
- Not surprisingly, due to the variance in LOS metrics and the per diem payment model, we also found a large variance in revenue among the hospitals, with the highest revenue hospital ($57,034) earning more than 3 times per case than the lowest revenue hospital ($16,149).
- Moreover, we found a significant correlation (R = 0.86 and R^2 = 0.74, p<0.01) between hospital LOS and hospital revenue for THR (Figure 7B).

Figure 6B: Distribution of THR hospital revenue

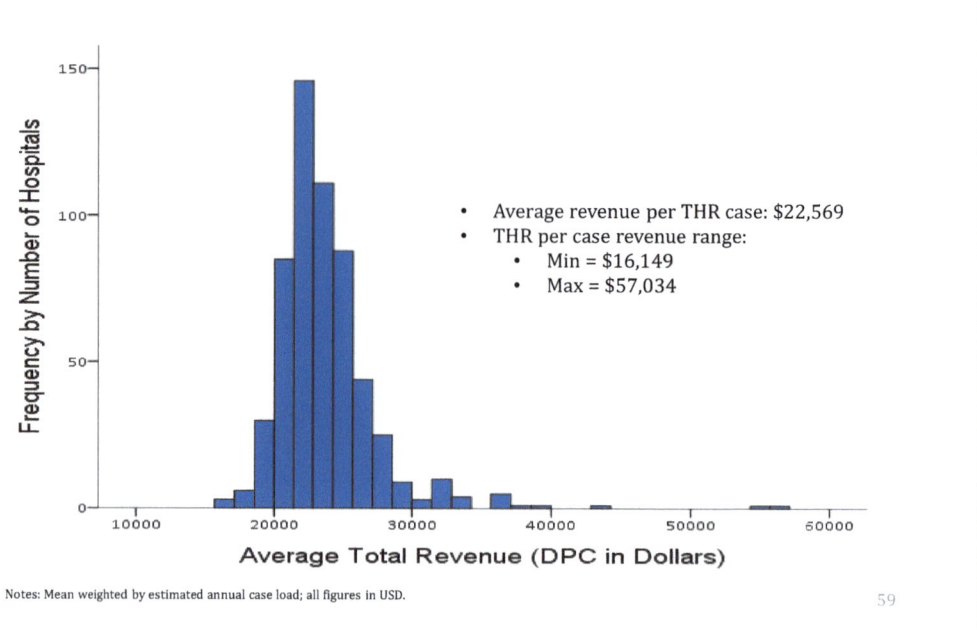

- Average revenue per THR case: $22,569
- THR per case revenue range:
  - Min = $16,149
  - Max = $57,034

Notes: Mean weighted by estimated annual case load; all figures in USD.

Figure 7B: THR hospital revenue per case vs. LOS

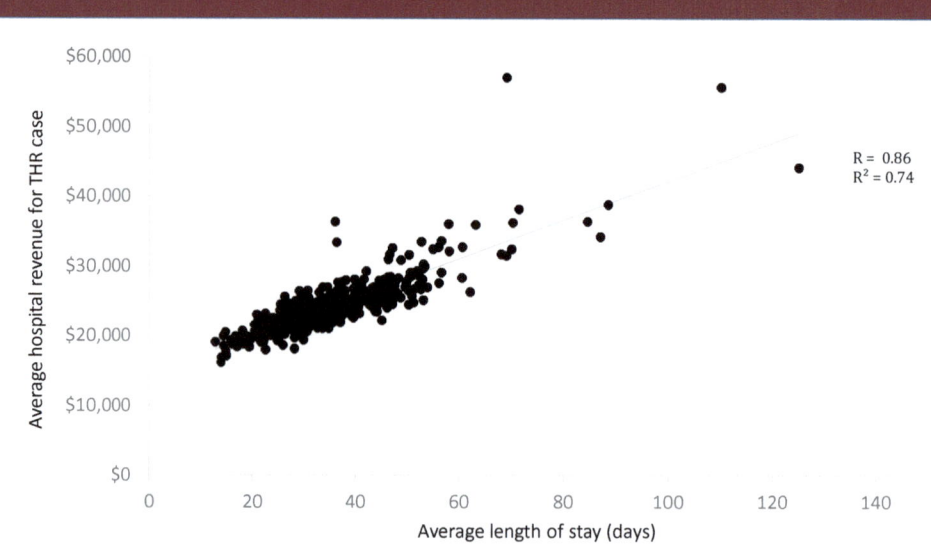

R = 0.86
R² = 0.74

Average length of stay is calculated across all cases of THR performed in a given facility and includes the acute portion of hospitalization only. Average hospital revenue is calculated by dividing the total DPC payments received by a facility by the total number of cases performed at that facility for the duration of observation. 574 DPC sample hospitals displayed and each point is representative of one hospital.

No clear relationship between hospital revenue per case and post-operative complications

- In contrast to the strong correlation observed for hospital revenue and LOS, we calculated R= 0.07, R^2 = 0.01 (p = 0.08) for the relationship between hospital revenue and post-operative complication rates.

- The average revenue per case is designated by the orange vertical line in Figure 8B and the orange horizontal line designates the average post-operative complication rate.

- Moreover, we found a large variation in revenue even for hospitals that had no post-surgical complications – from $16,149 to $38,775 per THR case (Figure 9B).

Figure 8B: THR post-operative complication rate vs. per case hospital revenue

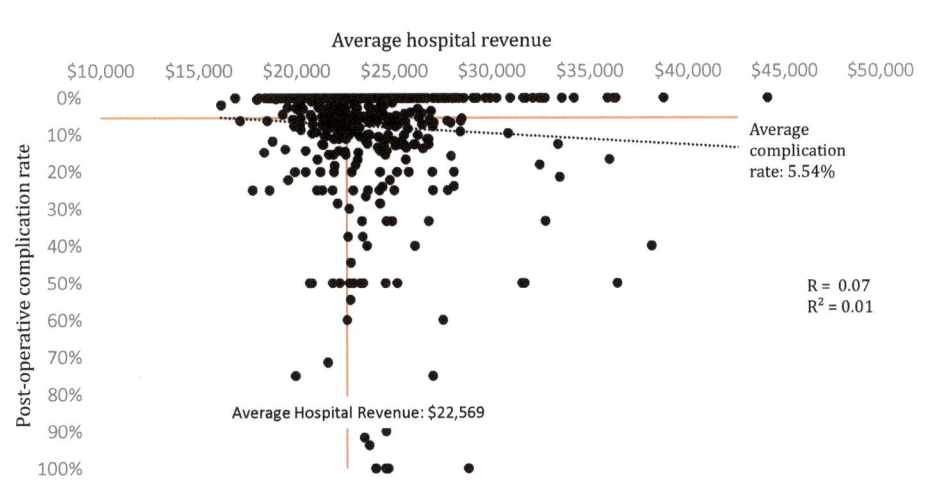

Post-operative complication rate is calculated for each facility and identified by one or more complication including surgical site infections, reoperation, post-op bleeding, post-op bed sores, post-op acute respiratory distress syndrome, pulmonary embolism, post-op septicemia, and in-hospital death. Average hospital revenue is calculated by dividing the total DPC payments received by a facility by the total number of cases performed at that facility for the duration of observation. Each point represents one hospital.

Figure 9B: Distribution of THR revenue per case in facilities with 0% post-operative complication rate

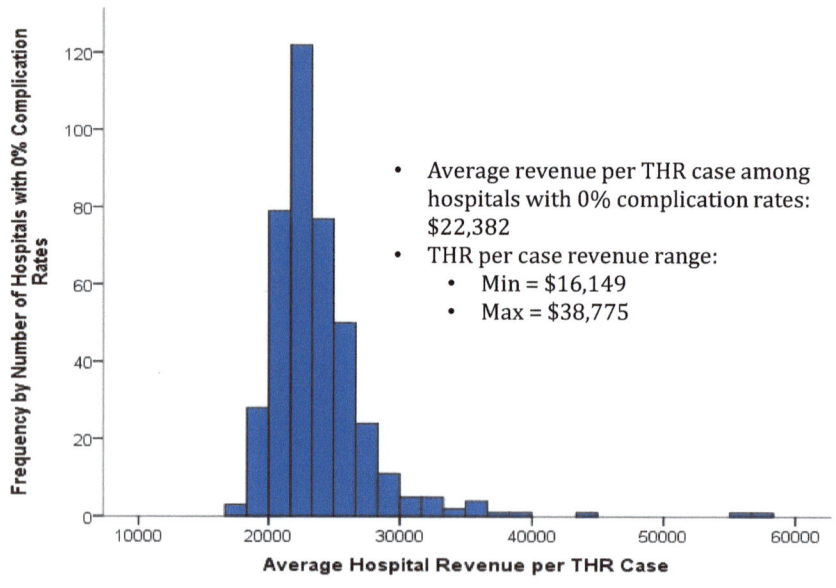

- Average revenue per THR case among hospitals with 0% complication rates: $22,382
- THR per case revenue range:
  - Min = $16,149
  - Max = $38,775

63

Discussion

Summary of findings

- On average, Japanese hospitals perform a lower annual volume of total joint replacements than U.S. hospitals, and complication rates tend to be higher in facilities with <70 annual total joint cases.

- We also found significant variability in quality and cost of care for total joint replacement in Japan. These observations hold true even for hospitals without post-operative complications. As a result there is a significant correlation between hospital length of stay and cost of care, but not complication rates.

- Although these findings may not be representative of the entire Japanese system (as they are limited to DPC hospitals and total joint procedures), they are nonetheless unexpected given the strong international reputation of the Japanese healthcare system.

- We hypothesize that variability in quality and cost of care is driven in part by the existing healthcare provider reimbursement structure.

U.S. studies have shown an inverse correlation between procedure volume and care quality

- When analyzing hip replacement procedures, Kreder and colleagues observed that "...patients managed by low-volume surgeons tended to have higher mortality rates, more infections, higher rates of revision operations, and more serious complications during the index hospitalization."[1]

- In turn, Hammond and colleagues analyzed 1,868 discrete total shoulder arthroplasties and hemiarthroplasties, concluding that "the risk of at least one complication associated with the procedures done by the high-volume surgeon group was nearly half that associated with the procedures done by the low-volume surgeon group."[2]

Source: 1) Kreder, HJ et al (1997). Relationship between the Volume of Total Hip Replacements Performed by Providers and the Rates of Postoperative Complications in the State of Washington. *The Journal of Bone and Joint Surgery*, 79(4):485-94; 2) Hammond, JW et al (2003). Surgeon experience and clinical and economic outcomes for shoulder arthroplasty. *The Journal of Bone and Joint Surgery*, 85: 2318-2324.

However, low surgical volumes may be a greater issue for Japan

- Although the correlation between low surgical volumes and higher complication rates is not unique to Japan, this may be a bigger issue for Japan than other countries due to the fact that 90% of our sample hospitals performed less than 70 total joint cases annually.

- Moreover, low case volumes have been observed among other surgical procedures in Japan:
  - "In a year, the average Japanese hospital performs only 107 percutaneous coronary interventions (PCI), the procedure that opens up blocked arteries, for example. This is half the volume that the American Heart Association and the American College of Cardiology recommend for good outcomes. (In other developed countries, the average number of PCIs per hospital ranges from 381 to 775.)"

- These observations may be related to the "relaxed" physician practice requirements that exist in Japan

Source: Henke, N et al (2009). Improving Japan's health care system. McKinsey & Company. http://www.mckinsey.com/insights/health_systems_and_services /improving_japans_health_care_system. Retrieved on: July 30, 2014.

Potential drivers of observed variation in hospital length of stay

- It is feasible that the observed differences in LOS are driven at least in part by the demographics of the patients in our hospital sample. Although, this may be true for TKR patients (median age in Japan of 75 years vs. 69 years in the U.S.), the THR patients in our hospital sample were actually slightly younger (median age of 67 years in Japan vs. 69 years in the U.S.).[1]

- One could also argue that the longer LOS observed in Japanese hospitals is a result of the observed post-operative complications, yet we found very little correlation between the post-operative complication rate of a given hospital and its patient LOS.

- In fact, the widest range in LOS for both procedures was observed in the subset of hospitals without any post-operative complications.

Source: Waddell, J; Johnson, K; Hein, W; Raabe, J; Fitzgerald, G; Turibio, F (2010). Orthopedic Practice in Total Hip and Total Knee Arthroplasty: Results From the Global Orthopaedic Registry (GLORY). *Am J Orthop*, 39(9 suppl):5-13.

Japan's per diem payment system promotes increased length of stay

- In a 2011 report from the Center for Strategic and International Studies, Anderson and Ikegami explored concerns raised by the Organization for Economic Cooperation and Development (OECD), the European Observatory, and McKinsey around the DPC hospital payment system. Among the concerns raised are the incentives created by the per diem payment model. [1]

- Under the DPC payment system, implemented in Japan in 2003, hospitals are reimbursed on a per diem basis, not a per case basis. Therefore, the underlying financial incentive is to extend a patient's length of stay within the hospital.

- Our data set seems to support these concerns as Japan remains a significant outlier internationally in terms of LOS for both procedures (29 days). In comparison, the median LOS for both procedures is 3 days in the U.S., 5 days in Canada, and 9 days in the UK.[2]

Source: 1) Anderson, G and N Ikegami (2011). *How Can Japan's DPC Inpatient Hospital Payment System Be Strengthened? Lessons from the U.S. Medicare Prospective System.* Center for Strategic and International Studies. http://csis.org/publication/how-can-japans-dpc-inpatient-hospital-payment-system-be-strengthened; 2) Waddell, J; Johnson, K; Hein, W; Raabe, J; Fitzgerald, G; Turibio, F (2010). Orthopedic Practice in Total Hip and Total Knee Arthroplasty: Results From the Global Orthopaedic Registry (GLORY). *Am J Orthop*, 39(9 suppl):5-13.

Outline

1. The Japanese healthcare system: Challenges and opportunities
2. Practice variation in Japan: Total joint replacements
3. Practice variation in the U.S.
4. Summary and Recommendations

71

- We have just shown that significant variability exists in care quality and expenditures for total joint replacement procedures in Japan.

- How does the U.S. compare and what are some potential lessons for providers and policy makers around the world on improving the value of healthcare delivery?

72

OECD finding of variability in quality and cost hold true for U.S. healthcare

- There is significant variability in healthcare value across the U.S. by medical center and geographic area, as measured by:
  - Mortality amenable to health care
  - Health care safety
  - Health care service
  - Mortality rates within teaching hospitals
  - Cost of care

The U.S. shows significant variability in patient outcomes

Mortality amenable to healthcare by state
Deaths per 100,000 population (2009-2010); OECD Average (2011)

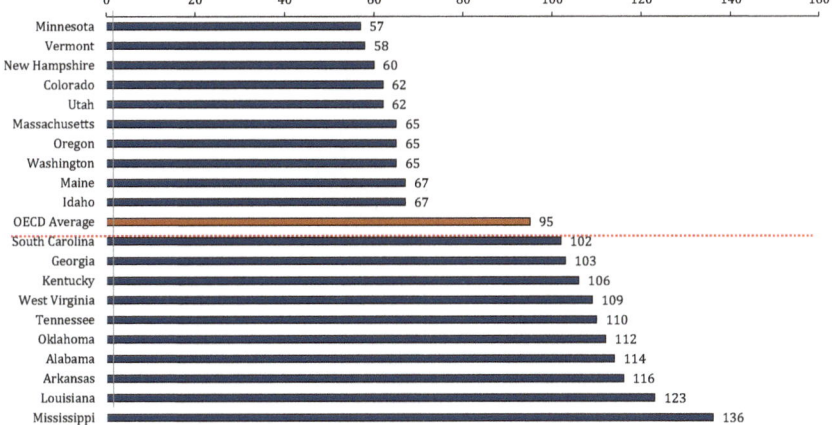

Notes: Mortality amenable to healthcare = Deaths before age 75 potentially preventable with timely and appropriate medical care. Only the top 10 and bottom 10 states are shown along with the OECD average.

Source: http://datacenter.commonwealthfund.org

Hospital safety measures also vary widely across the U.S.

Percent of hospitals receiving the top safety rating (A) by state (2011-2012)

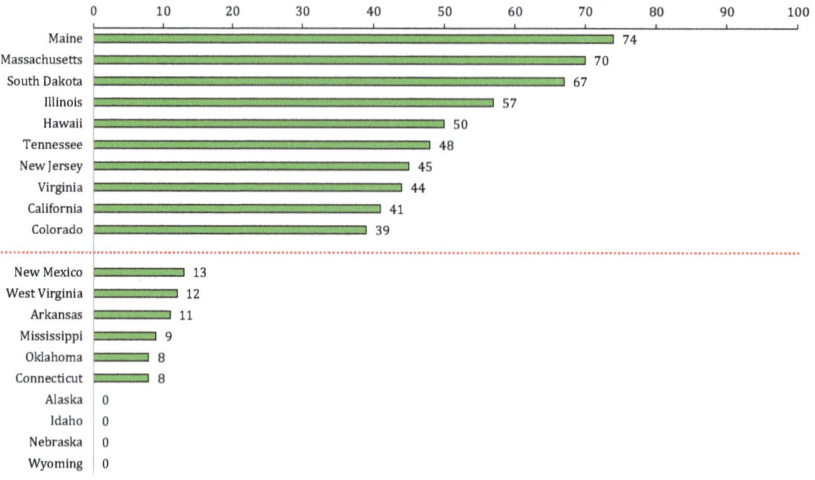

Notes: Only the top 10 and bottom 10 states are shown.

Source: http://www.hospitalsafetyscore.org/state-rankings; https://data.medicare.gov/Hospital-Compare/Survey-of-Patients-Hospital-ExperiencesHCAHPS-Sta/fhk8-g4vc

75

Patient satisfaction also varies widely across the U.S.

Percent of patients who 'would definitely recommend the hospital' by state (July 2011-June 2012)

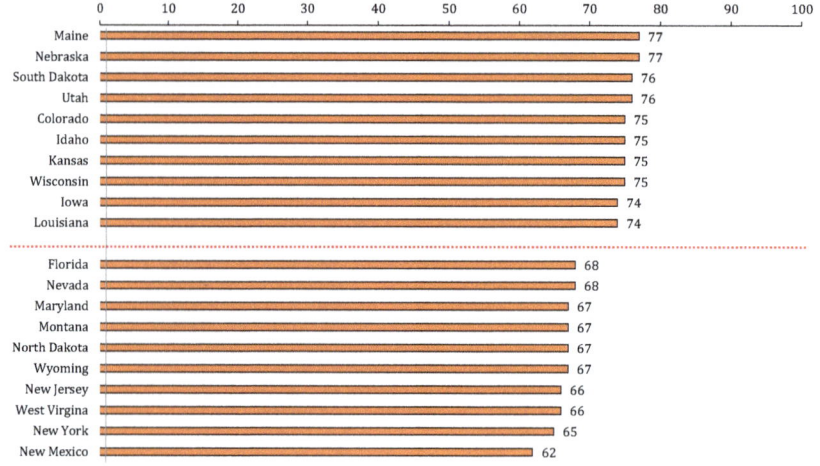

Notes: Only the top 10 and bottom 10 states are shown.

Source: https://data.medicare.gov/data/hospital-compare

76

Due to their unique access to the latest technology and use of best clinical practices, one would expect that teaching hospitals would produce consistent and positive patient outcomes.

However, even teaching hospitals show wide variability in outcomes

Variability in mortality ratios among COTH hospitals in the U.S. (2009)

COTH hospitals	**Mortality ratio** >1.0 = better than expected
Best hospital in category	2.06
Worst hospital in category	0.65
Teaching hospital average	**1.02**

Notes: The mean for all teaching hospitals is 1.02. The best hospital scored 2.06, or over 100% better than expected. While the worst hospital scored 0.65, 35% worse than expected. COTH = Council of Teaching Hospitals and Health Systems; n = 269 COTH member facilities (excludes COTH member VA and Children's hospitals, as well as facilities with <50 actual deaths in 2009; Mortality ratio for each facility is calculated as expected deaths/ observed deaths in a given year.

Source: "Council of Teaching Hospitals and Health Systems – Member Communities – AAMC." Accessed June 2011. https://www.aamc.org/members/coth/; Medicare Provider Analysis and Review (MedPar) file 2009 (Accessed July 2011).

The U.S. also shows significant variability in the cost of healthcare

Medicare fee-for-service spending by hospital referral region (2008)

Geographic region	Average standardized risk-adjusted per capita costs ($USD)	Ratio to benchmark (national average)
Lowest cost 10% of providers	$6,194	0.8
Lowest cost 20% of providers	$6,613	0.9
National average	$7,500	Benchmark
Highest cost 20% of providers	$8,301	1.1
Highest cost 10% of providers	$8,849	1.2

Notes: Total = National average standardized risk adjusted per capita cost x total Medicare beneficiaries in sample; Total Medicare beneficiaries n = 25,832,920; Standardization of Spending: To standardize payment rates, examined Medicare's various FFS payment systems and identified the factors that lead to different payment rates for the same service (e.g., local wages, input prices, DSH, GME); Estimated what Medicare would have paid for each claim without those adjustments; Risk-Adjustment of Spending: Used total Hierarchical Condition Category (HCC) risk scores to risk-adjust spending data; Calculated standardized risk-adjusted costs by taking the standardized costs for each beneficiary in a region and dividing them by his/her actual individual risk score. National average includes VI, PR, DC and unassigned data

Source: Institute of Medicine. 2011. "New Data on Geographic Variation." http://iom.edu/Activities/HealthServices/GeographicVariation/Data-Resources.aspx.

Total joint procedures in the U.S. reveal a similar degree of variability as Japan

- "The study showed substantial variations across the participating health care organizations in surgery times, hospital lengths-of-stay, discharge dispositions, and in-hospital complication rates.

- The study also revealed that higher surgeon caseloads were associated with shorter lengths-of-stay and operating time, as well as fewer in-hospital complications."

Source: Tomek et al. 2012. A Collaborative Of Leading Health Systems Finds Wide Variations In Total Knee Replacement Delivery And Takes Steps To Improve Value. *Health Affairs* 31(6):1329-38. doi: 10.1377/hlthaff.2011.0935.

Outline

1. The Japanese healthcare system: Challenges and opportunities
2. Practice variation in Japan: Total joint replacements
3. Practice variation in the U.S.
4. Summary and Recommendations

81

Summary

- We hypothesize that the current payment structures, in both the U.S. and Japan, are contributing to the variability in value we are experiencing among healthcare providers working within these systems.

- Providers in both countries receive financial compensation without any reference to the quality of care or overall care efficiency.

- Instead, the recently introduced DPC graduated per diem payment mechanism in Japan, provides financial incentive for long lengths of stay and likely leads to increasing patient complications.

- Meanwhile the U.S. DRG payment system, which only includes hospital services and not physician fees, fails to promote value and lacks any incentive to coordinate care among providers.

82

Experts agree that in order to reduce
variability in quality and cost to improve value,
we need to address systems incentives…

U.S. provider reimbursement mechanisms create limited incentives to deliver high-value care (1/2)

- The predominant fee-for-service (FFS) payment
  mechanism reimburses physicians based on per-unit-of-
  service without any reference to the quality (outcomes,
  safety, service) of care received.
- Moreover, the low levels of reimbursement and per-unit-
  of-service price controls imposed by government payers
  have created a system that incentivizes the overuse of
  services and procedures.

U.S. provider reimbursement mechanisms create limited incentives to deliver high-value care (2/2)

- Furthermore, payments are delivered in silos and often with conflicting incentives:
  - Hospitals: Diagnosis related groups (DRGs)
  - Nursing homes: Per diem
  - Physicians: Fee-for-service
- This constellation of factors creates limited financial incentives for the various parts of the care system to work together to create better value.

The Japanese provider reimbursement system does not fare any better than the U.S.

- In Japan, the DPC, per diem graduated payment system incentivizes and, as supported by our data, results in prolonged length of stays.
- Additionally, Japanese physicians work under a fee-for-service reimbursement model which further incentivizes overutilization.
- All of these payment systems fail to promote value, collaboration, and integration.

All participants in the healthcare delivery system should be paid for value

- This means that payments would be linked to quality and total cost of care, not just compliance with a certain pre-determined process.
- Building the value equation into the reimbursement model inherently creates the need for collaboration among various providers, administrative staff, and caregivers in order to determine the best treatment plan for the patient.
- Collaborative efforts under this model have unprecedented potential for quality of care as for the first time, underlying incentives will be aligned across the industry.

87

"Since value depends on results, not inputs, value in healthcare is measured by the outcomes achieved, not the volume of services delivered, and shifting focus from volume to value is a central challenge."

- Michael Porter, PhD

What do we mean by pay-for-value?

- In the simplest of terms, paying-for-value means that reimbursements are linked directly to what is delivered.
- In order to truly pay-for-value, reimbursement needs to be linked to the quality of care and overall treatment costs.

Moving towards paying-for-value

- The majority of current payment schemes are not tied to quality or to total cost of care.
- For example, in the U.S. attempts to institute "pay for performance" schemes have fallen short of true "pay for value" because *performance* has been equated with *compliance with process* – rather than with quality of care.

Current Pay for Performance (P4P) approaches are not necessarily Pay for Value, but rather Pay for Compliance

"These current [P4P] efforts…carry some risks. Most…are not actually about quality results, but processes. Most 'pay for performance' is really pay for compliance. Compliance to too many process standards…runs the risk of inhibiting innovation by the best providers."

Michael Porter and Elizabeth Teisberg

Notes: Pay for performance is a payment scheme in which a portion of the payment is based on performance assessed against a defined measure.

Source: Porter, Michael E., and Elizabeth Olmsted Teisberg. 2006. *Redefining Health Care: Creating Value-Based Competition on Results*. Boston: Harvard Business School Press.

- As Porter and Teisberg point out, we should concentrate on quality, not process.
- So take the case of two California metropolitan teaching hospitals that treat similar Medicare patients.
- Assume both complete the P4P Medicare processes and receive a 5% P4P bonus.

P4P bonus structure actually pays for lower efficiency... and worse outcomes!

Patient outcomes and costs within two California teaching hospitals*

	Medical Center A	Medical Center B
Care efficiency (utilization & cost)		
• Hospital days per patient	11.1	23.0
• Physician visits per patient	35.5	81.8
• Total Medicare reimbursement per patient ($000)	$37.0	$62.2
Care effectiveness (outcomes)		
• Mortality ratio (>1 = better than expected)	1.43	0.88
5% P4P bonus	**$1,851**	**$3,112**

Note that in this example, using real data, under a P4P system rewarding medical centers on process items, the worst mortality rate medical center would get the highest reward.

*All data are for Medicare beneficiaries, last 6 months of life; data from two prominent teaching hospitals in CA.
Source: The Dartmouth Atlas of Health Care (accessed May 25, 2011), http://www.dartmouthatlas.org/data/topic/; Medicare Provider Analysis and Review (MedPar) file 2009 (Accessed July 2011).

In fact, P4P process metrics bring few – if any – gains in patient outcomes.

- "Among hospitals participating in a voluntary quality-improvement initiative, the pay-for-performance program was not associated with a significant incremental improvement in quality of care or outcomes for acute myocardial infarction."[1]

- "We are aware that improvements in process measures do not necessarily translate into improved clinical outcomes. As illustrated by our results, it is much easier to make sure a patient with diabetes received a [cholesterol] order each year, than it is to ensure that the [cholesterol] is controlled to appropriate levels."[2]

- "Our analysis...demonstrates that the current generation of P4P measures based on process is inadequate. Hospital quality measures did not correlate with complications or mortality."[3]

Source: 1) Glickman et al. 2007. "Pay for Performance, Quality of Care, and Outcomes in Acute Myocardial Infarction." *JAMA* 297(21):2373-2380; 2) Weber et al. 2008. "Employing the Electronic Health Record to Improve Diabetes Care: A Multifaceted Intervention in an Integrated Delivery System." *J Gen Intern Med* 23(4):379–382; 3) Bhattacharyya et al. 2009. "Measuring the Report Card: The Validity of Pay-For-Performance Metrics in Orthopedic Surgery." *Health Affairs* 28(2):526-532.

Moreover, compliance with process has the potential to stifle clinical innovation

A number of clinical processes widely accepted in the past have seen significant revisions in current medical practice, e.g.,

- Bed rest of 3-6 weeks, previously a standard of care following an episode of acute myocardial infarction (AMI), has been shown to be not only unnecessary but potentially harmful to AMI patients.[1]

- Beta-blockers, that were absolutely contraindicated in patients with congestive heart failure (CHF), are now considered to be standard of care and a key component of the medication regimen in CHF treatment.[2]

Source: 1) Allen et al. 1999. "Bed Rest: A Potentially Harmful Treatment Needing More Careful Evaluation." *Lancet* 354(9186):1229-33; 2) Packer et al. 1996. "The Effect of Carvedilol on Morbidity and Mortality in Patients with Chronic Heart Failure." *NEJM* 334:1349-1355.

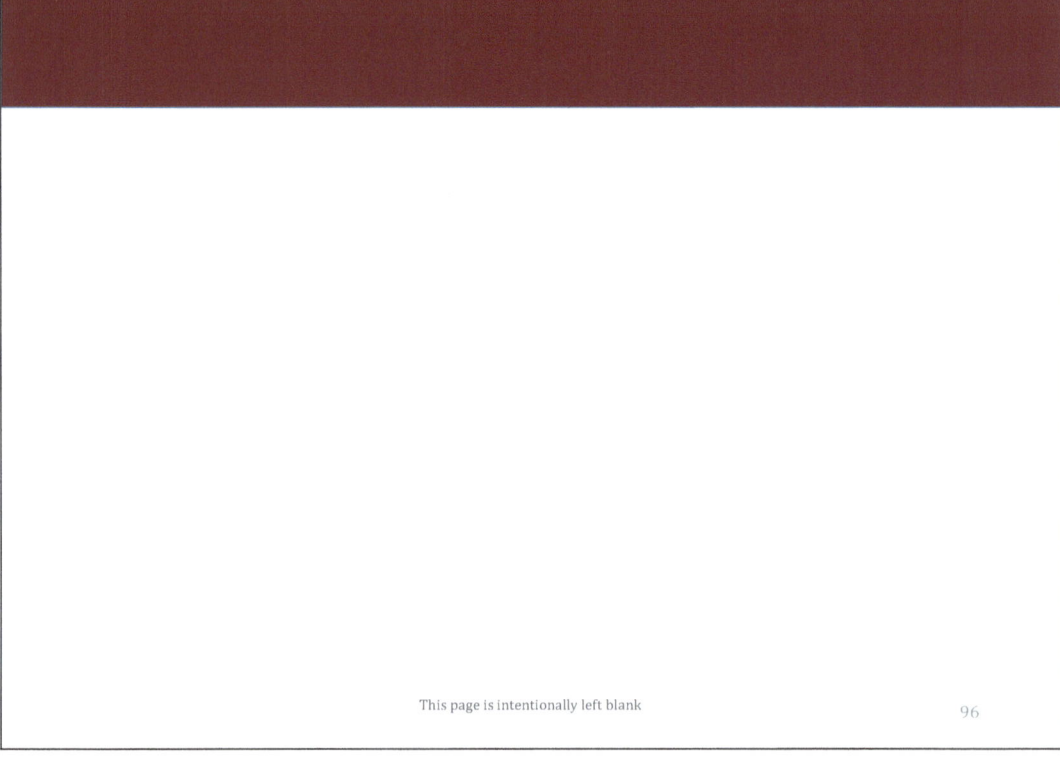

Recommendations

- We need a new payment approach, one that focuses on paying-for-value measured by quality of care and total treatment costs.
- A payment approach that is not simply based upon adherence to process measures.
- In order to properly structure a system where provider incentives are aligned to value and not volume, we propose that both the U.S. and Japan move to an Expanded Diagnosis Related Group (EDRG) payment system.

What is an EDRG?

- Just as the name suggests, an EDRG is an extension of the already existing U.S. DRG payment model.
- It would contain much of the same elements that exist within the DRG model including bundled payments for various procedures.
- However unlike the current models, EDRG's hold the potential pathway to a pay-for-value system by expanding to include:
  - Physician services, and
  - All services related to the procedure occurring within a pre-defined period following admission (e.g., 30, 60, or 90 days post-admission).

"The idea is to force all of a patient's care providers to work together. They have a strong incentive to eliminate unnecessary tests and treatments and use less expensive implants, drugs, and devices that don't compromise quality, and to prevent infections and other complications that could land the patient back in the hospital."

- Dr. Ezekiel J. Emanuel

Source: Ezekiel J. Emanuel, "Saving by the Bundle," New York Times, November 16, 2011.

Why EDRGs and why now (1/3)

- Collaboration among providers is an essential element to effectively restructure the healthcare system to deliver high-value care.
- Implementing EDRG payments will serve as a forcing function for various providers to work in a more integrated fashion.
- Furthermore, since their incentives would be aligned to produce better quality at lower costs, it is in everyone's best interest to ensure that variability is reduced, and in turn best practices are developed and utilized.

Why EDRGs and why now (2/3)

- If successful, these providers will also be in a much better position to assume increased responsibility, accountability, and authority in the care of patients.
- We recognize many experts strongly support full capitation as the best way to reward value. But most providers are not yet equipped with some of the elements necessary to handle the demands full capitation could create.

Why EDRGs and why now (3/3)

- The integration, infrastructure, and best practices that will be developed in order to succeed under EDRG payments, will in turn, support the management of patients under larger models of bundled payments and full capitation.
- Therefore, using EDRGs to build upon the already familiar DRG model is a good starting point for aligning providers on the path to further reform.

Where to start with EDRGs?

1. Determine the most expensive DRGs/DPCs and create an EDRG for those conditions or procedures.

2. Use lump-sum (bundled) payments to establish EDRGs, and thus encourage judicious use rates.

3. Define quality, not process metrics.

4. Give providers two to three years to self-organize for EDRGs. Experience with standard DRGs over the past 25 years has proven this can be done successfully.

Identify and address the highest cost patients

- One way to restrain overall healthcare costs is to concentrate efforts on the small percent of the population that drives the majority of the costs – rather than focusing efforts on the vast majority of the population that accounts for only a small share of the overall costs (see next slide).

- For example, in the U.S. the majority of the highest cost Medicare patients are the sickest patients who end up being hospitalized for their conditions.

- Payment approaches providing incentives for more integrated and coordinated care, hold the potential to reduce the extensive use of resources and their associated costs that these sick patients require.

- Instead, the incentive will then be to ensure that the patients have the resources and education necessary to remain healthy, at home, and out of the hospital.

In any given year, 20% of the population accounts for 80% of total healthcare spending

Concentration of healthcare spending in the U.S. population (2009)

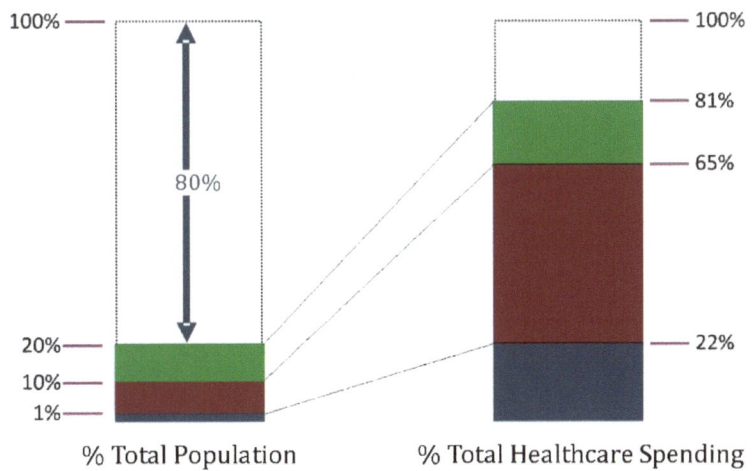

% Total Population   % Total Healthcare Spending

Source: "Health Care Costs: A Primer - Kaiser Family Foundation." Accessed May 17, 2012. http://www.kff.org/insurance/7670.cfm

105

Where to start with EDRGs?

1. Determine the most expensive DRGs/DPCs and create an EDRG for those conditions or procedures.

2. Use lump-sum (bundled) payments to establish EDRGs, and thus encourage judicious use rates.

3. Define quality, not process metrics.

4. Give providers two to three years to self-organize for EDRGs. Experience with standard DRGs over the past 25 years has proven this can be done successfully.

106

One bundled payment for:

Hospital Services

+

Post-discharge care

+

Physician services related to medical
condition for a specified period of time

Expanded DRG

Where to start with EDRGs?

1. Determine the most expensive DRGs/DPCs and create
   an EDRG for those conditions or procedures.
2. Use lump-sum (bundled) payments to establish EDRGs,
   and thus encourage judicious use rates.
3. Define quality, not process metrics.
4. Give providers two to three years to self-organize for
   EDRGs. Experience with standard DRGs over the past
   25 years has proven this can be done successfully.

True pay-for-value means tying payments to quality and cost over time

- These quality metrics should be condition or DRG specific.
- Quality measures and post-admission time frames should be set by the physicians treating each particular disease category (e.g., orthopedic surgeons would determine outcomes to track for total joint patients).
- Favor independent or private oversight of quality measurements, because:
  - Government efforts are often subject to politics and lobbying.
  - Government defined quality metrics tend to be watered down and turned into process measures.

Where to start with EDRGs?

1. Determine the most expensive DRGs/DPCs and create an EDRG for those conditions or procedures.
2. Use lump-sum (bundled) payments to establish EDRGs, and thus encourage judicious use rates.
3. Define quality, not process metrics.
4. Give providers two to three years to self-organize for EDRGs. Experience with standard DRGs over the past 25 years has proven this can be done successfully.

Will this not result in increased utilization?

- The widely held expectations surrounding the DRG payment model, namely
  - Increase in hospital efficiency (by reducing length of stay), but also
  - Increase in total case volume
- Did not come true in the U.S., as highlighted in the next slide.

Source: Street A, O'Reilly J, Ward P, Mason A. DRG-based hospital payment and efficiency: theory, evidence, and challenges. In: Busse R, Geissler A, Quentin W, Wiley M, editors. *Diagnosis-related groups in Europe: moving towards transparency, efficiency and quality in hospitals.* Maidenhead: Open University Press; 2011. pp. 93–114.

The introduction of DRGs resulted in reduced utilization of healthcare services

Change in utilization of healthcare services pre and post DRG introduction
Percent

Metric	Pre-DRG (1980-1985)	Post-DRG (1988-1992)	Percent change
Average length of stay (days)	6.9	6.4	-8%
Hospital admissions (per 1,000 population)	163	125	-23%
Hospital days (per 1,000 population)	1,129	800	-29%

Source: Department of Health & Human Services, Centers for Disease Control and Prevention. 1989. "Trends in Hospital Utilization: United States,1965-1986. Data from the National Health Survey." Series 13, Number 101; Department of Health & Human Services, Centers for Disease Control and Prevention. 1996. "Trends in Hospital Utilization: United States, 1988-92. Data From the National Health Survey." Series 13, number 124. http://www.cdc.gov/nchs/nhds.htm.

Setting the base EDRG payment amount

- Do not use complex formulas
- Instead, use reality-based pricing. For example, the base payment amount could be set at the 75th percentile of the high value quadrant medical centers, i.e., hospitals that get better than average quality at lower than average total cost per case.
- The following figure shows an example distribution of Japanese hospitals by both quality and cost per case. The high value medical center quadrant is outlined in this graph.

Notes: Total cost per case to the payer = hospital revenue/ case

113

Distribution of outcomes and costs for TKR in our hospital sample

TKR post-operative complications vs. hospital revenue

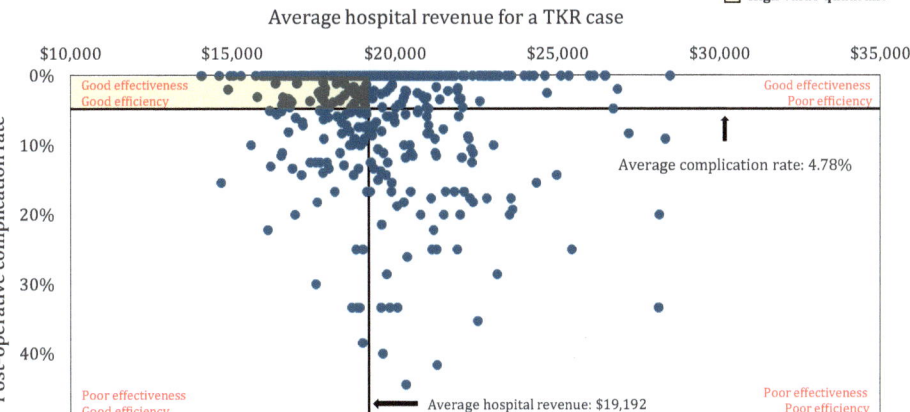

Post-operative complication rate is calculated for each facility and identified by one or more complication including surgical site infections, reoperation, post-op bleeding, post-op bed sores, post-op acute respiratory distress syndrome, pulmonary embolism, post-op septicemia, and in-hospital death. Average hospital revenue is calculated by dividing the total DPC payments received by a facility by the total number of cases performed at that facility for the duration of observation. Each point represents one hospital. Hospitals with >50% complication rate not shown.

114

Building in financial incentives to improve quality

- Setting the EDRG payment amount at the 75th percentile of hospitals in the high value quadrant encourages efficiency by all hospitals. But it also allows hospitals in the lower left quadrant (good efficiency, but poor quality) to do well financially.

- To provide an incentive for both efficiency and better quality, we would suggest that a quality withhold of 5% be established. If a medical center's quality is not at least as good as the average hospital quality metrics, those hospitals would receive 5% less than the target amount, or $17,744 (1,792,297 J Yen) in our example (see next slide).

- Thus, all hospitals in the two upper quadrants would receive a single bundled payment of $18,678 (1,886,628 J Yen), while the hospitals in the lower quadrants would receive $17,744 (1,792,297 J Yen). The 5% withhold may be reversed, if in the subsequent years, the hospital in question is able improve its quality.

To ensure that we do not sacrifice quality for cost with EDRGs, a quality withhold approach may be warranted

TKR post-operative complications vs. hospital revenue

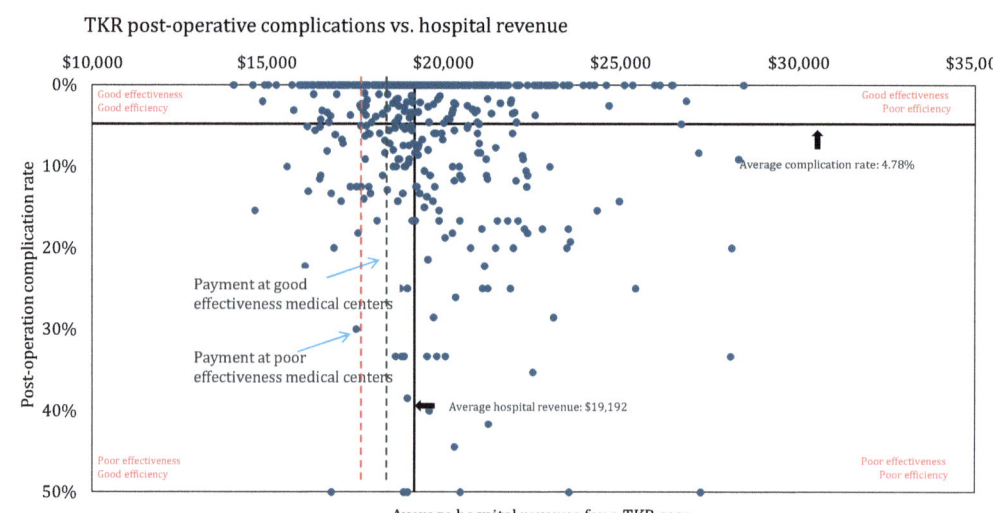

Post-operative complication rate is calculated for each facility and identified by one or more complication including surgical site infections, reoperation, post-op bleeding, post-op bed sores, post-op acute respiratory distress syndrome, pulmonary embolism, post-op septicemia, and in-hospital death. Average hospital revenue is calculated by dividing the total DPC payments received by a facility by the total number of cases performed at that facility for the duration of observation. Each point represents one hospital. Hospitals with >50% complication rate not shown.

Has anyone actually implemented a payment scheme like EDRGs? What was the result?

"EDRG" type payment for hip and knee replacement in Stockholm, Sweden

- Components of the bundle

• Pre-op evaluation	• Physicians fees
• Lab tests	• Any additional surgery to the joint within 2 years
• Radiology	
• Surgery	• If post-op infection requiring antibiotics occurs, guarantee extends to 5 years
• Prothesis	
• Drugs	
• Rehabilitation	

- 3.2% quality withhold

- Data on 3 years post implementation

Source: Porter, Michael, E. "Value-based healthcare delivery: reimbursement. *Harvard Business School: Institute for Strategy and Competitiveness*. 2012.
http://www.hbs.edu/faculty/Publication%20Files/Reimbursement%20Intensive%20Seminar%202012_230391a3-3491-4d26-b8fb-88e550a93a84.pdf.

In Sweden, "EDRG" type reimbursement improved quality

Post-surgical complications

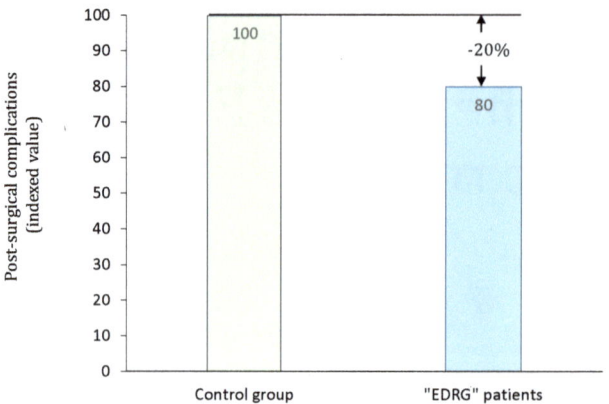

Source: Clawson et al (2014). "Competing on outcomes: winning strategies for value-based healthcare. *The Boston Consulting Group*. 2014.
https://www.bcgperspectives.com/content/articles/health_care_payers_providers_biopharma_competing_on_outcomes_winning_strategies_value_b
ased_health_care/c

In Sweden, "EDRG" type reimbursement also reduced cost

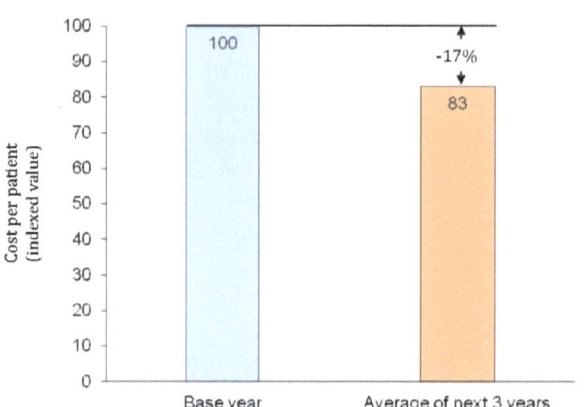

Source: Clawson et al (2014). "Competing on outcomes: winning strategies for value-based healthcare. *The Boston Consulting Group*. 2014.
https://www.bcgperspectives.com/content/articles/health_care_payers_providers_biopharma_competing_on_outcomes_winning_strategies_value_b
ased_health_care/c

Care delivery changes by Swedish medical centers with "EDRG" type payments

- Explicit care pathways
- Standardized treatment processes
- Checklists
- New post-discharge visit to check would healing

- More patient education
- More training and specialization of staff
- Increased procedures per day
- Decreased length of stay

Source: Porter, Michael, E. "Value-based healthcare delivery: reimbursement. *Harvard Business School: Institute for Strategy and Competitiveness.* 2012.
http://www.hbs.edu/faculty/Publication%20Files/Reimbursement%20Intensive%20Seminar%202012_230391a3-3491-4d26-b8fb-88e550a93a84.pdf

Sweden's expansion of "ERDG" type pricing

- Spine surgery added September 2013.
- Increased quality withhold to 10% from 3.2%.
- 8 additional medical conditions to be added in 2015.

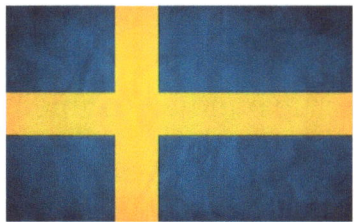

Source: Clawson et al (2014). "Competing on outcomes: winning strategies for value-based healthcare. *The Boston Consulting Group.* 2014.
https://www.bcgperspectives.com/content/articles/health_care_payers_providers_biopharma_competing_on_outcomes_winning_strategies_value_based_health_care/c

- EDRG results from Sweden suggest that using a bundled-payment approach to enhance value has "universal" applicability.
- While the details of implementation may vary, we believe that the basic principles apply even in settings as different in organization and culture as the healthcare sectors in the US and Japan.

Conclusions

- All countries say they would like to have higher value healthcare. But for the most part these countries are wishing for a better result while basically continuing to do things as they have in the past.
- If we want high value healthcare, we are more likely to get it if we actually start paying for it. Thus, we need a new payment approach, one that focuses on paying-for-value measured by quality of care and total treatment costs.
- By establishing a true bundled payment with a quality withhold (in the manner described above) the payers can take one more step toward creating the right sets of incentives to promote higher value healthcare.

So, if we could do just one thing...

- **Change existing financial incentives and start paying for value:** Set payment based on care quality and true cost of care by establishing Expanded DRGs.

- If we accomplish this correctly, providers will self-organize into systems that produce high-value care.

About the authors

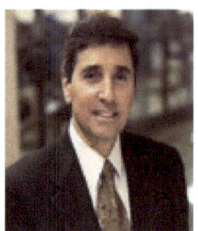

Denis A. Cortese, MD
Dr. Cortese's current positions include Foundation Professor at Arizona State University (ASU), Director of ASU's Healthcare Delivery and Policy Program, and President of the non-profit Healthcare Transformation Institute based in Phoenix, AZ. He is an Emeritus President and CEO of the Mayo Clinic. Dr. Cortese also currently serves on the board of trustees of Dartmouth-Hitchcock, and the boards of directors for Cerner Corporation, Essence Global Holding Corporation, and Pinnacle West. Memberships in national and international organizations include: the Institute of Medicine of the National Academy of Sciences, where he served as the original chair of the Roundtable on Value and Science-Driven Health Care; a National Associate of the National Research Council; an honorary member of the Royal College of Physicians (London) and the Academia Nacional de Medicina (Mexico). He formerly served in the following positions: member of the health advisory board of RAND; member, and served as the chair of the board, of the Health Care Leadership Council in Washington, DC.; member of the Harvard/Kennedy Health Policy Group; member of the Division on Engineering and Physical Science (DEPS) of the National Academy of Engineering. Education includes a BS from Franklin and Marshall, an MD from Temple University, and residency training in Internal Medicine and Pulmonary Diseases at the Mayo Clinic. Awards include an Ellis Island Award in 2007 and the National Healthcare Leadership Award in 2009.

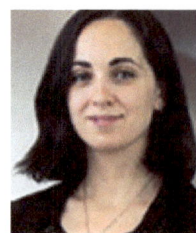

Natalie Landman, PhD
Dr. Natalie Landman is currently the Associate Director for Projects at the ASU Healthcare Delivery and Policy Program (HCDPP). In this role, Natalie is responsible for managing the portfolio of HCDPP projects, including project definition, launch, and implementation, as well as serving as a liaison to academic, private, government, and non-profit entities in support of HCDPP mission. Natalie joined ASU after nearly three years at McKinsey & Company, where she served numerous clients in the healthcare and high tech sectors on a range of strategic topics including business unit and corporate growth strategy, product development, marketing and brand management. Natalie holds a PhD in Neurobiology and Behavior from Columbia University in New York City. While at Columbia, Natalie also served on the R&D and Business Development teams of SMART Biosciences, Inc., a Columbia spin-off biotechnology company with technology platforms in Alzheimer's disease and oncology.

About the authors

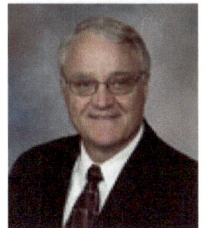

Robert K. Smoldt, MBA
Mr. Smoldt is Chief Administrative Officer Emeritus of the Mayo Clinic. He served as a member of the Mayo Clinic Board of Trustees and Mayo Clinic Executive Committee from 1990 through 2007, and is presently the Director of the ASU Healthcare Delivery and Policy Program. Mr Smoldt served two terms on the Board of Catholic Health Initiatives and continues as a member of its Finance Committee. Mr. Smoldt earned a BS from Iowa State University and an MBA from the University of Southern California. He has given numerous presentations and is a recognized speaker on the healthcare environment. Mr. Smoldt has been involved in healthcare administration for over 30 years — both with the U.S. Air Force and the Mayo Clinic. Mr. Smoldt has also been active in the Medical Group Management Association. He has chaired the organization's research and marketing committees and has acted as moderator of its international conference in London, UK. Most recently, he was a member of the Medical Group Management Association National Awards Committee, which honors those who make significant leadership contributions to healthcare administration. In January 2010 Mr. Smoldt accepted the position of Associate Director of Arizona State University's Healthcare Delivery and Policy Program.

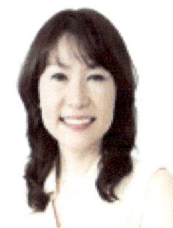

Sachiko Watanabe, RN, MHSA, MAE
Ms. Watanabe is the CEO of the Global Health Consulting Japan (GHC). Ms. Watanabe, originally trained as a nurse, graduated from the Keio University majoring in economics and also earned two master's degrees from University of Michigan. GHC is a rapidly growing consulting firm specializing in hospital managements in Japan. Under Ms. Watanabe's leadership, GHC has grown to be the top hospital management consulting firm in Japan and provides management and benchmark services to over 800 major hospitals. She is a well-known author and a commentator in health related issues in Japan.

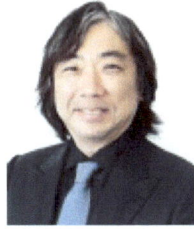

Aki Yoshikawa, PhD
Dr. Aki Yoshikawa is the chairman of the Global Health Consulting. Before joining the GHC, Dr. Yoshikawa, a Berkeley educated health economist, directed the Comparative Health Care Policy Research Project at Stanford University. He is an author of Health Economics of Japan: Patients, Doctors, and Hospitals under a Universal Health Insurance System (University or Tokyo Press, 1996), and Japan's Health System: Efficiency and Effectiveness in Universal Care (Faulkner & Gray, 1993). He has published more than 100 academic articles.

www.ingramcontent.com/pod-product-compliance
Lightning Source LLC
Chambersburg PA
CBHW050742180526
45159CB00003B/1323

* 9 7 8 1 5 1 7 3 8 3 8 5 5 *